Beating
Cancer with
Natural
Medicine

Michael Lam, MD

ISBN: 1-4107-3244-4 (e-book)
ISBN: 1-4107-3243-6 (Paperback)
ISBN: 1-4107-3242-8 (Hardcover)

Library of Congress Control Number: 2003094823

This book is printed on acid free paper.

Printed in the United States of America
Bloomington, IN

1stBooks – rev. 06/30/03

ABOUT THE AUTHOR

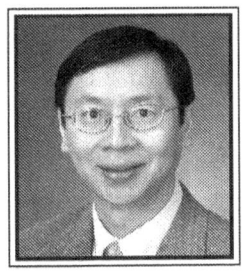 **Michael Lam, MD, MPH, ABAAM, CNC** is a specialist in Nutritional and Anti-Aging Medicine. He is currently the Director of Medical Education at the Academy of Anti-Aging Research, USA, overseeing the global education program for physicians and researchers in this field. Dr Lam received his Bachelor of Science degree from Oregon State University and his Doctor of Medicine degree from Loma Linda University School of Medicine, California. He also holds a Masters of Public Health degree in Preventive Health, and is Board Certified by the American Board of Anti-aging Medicine. Dr Lam is credited for being the first to formulate the three clinical phases of aging, and is a pioneer in using non-toxic natural compounds to treat age related degenerative diseases. His clinical specialty focuses on the use of optimum blends of nutritional supplementation that manipulates food, vitamins, natural hormones, herbs, enzymes, and mineral into specific protocols to rejuvenate cellular function. He is a recognized expert in nutritional medicine, being a Certified Nutritional Consultant and a Diplomat of the American Association of Nutritional Consultants. Dr Lam has been published extensively in this field. He has written over 50 articles on natural medicine and the books *The Five Proven Secrets to Longevity* and *How to Stay Young and Live Longer*. He is listed in the International Who's Who of Professionals, serves as editor of the Journal of Anti-Aging Research, and is a Board Examiner for the American Academy of Anti-Aging Medicine.

To learn more about nutritional and anti-aging medicine, visit Dr Lam's public education website (www.LamMD.com).

CONTENTS

INTRODUCTION	**9**
EXECUTIVE SUMMARY	**14**
War On Cancer	14
Cancer – According to Natural Medicine	15
The rate of success	16
Know your enemy	17
Natural Medicine – Your Choice	19
7 Steps To Beating Cancer Naturally	21
General Cancer Nutraceutical Model	23
Conclusion	26

CHAPTER ONE

MY DOCTOR IS KILLING ME!	**29**
How Good Is Your Healthcare?	32
Adult Cancer – A Degenerative Disease?	35
Conventional Therapies – Hitting A Plateau	40
Surgery (Cut)	41
Chemotherapy (Poison)	41
Radiation therapy (Burn)	44
Side effects	44
War on Cancer – Who is Winning?	46
Natural vs. Conventional Medicine	48
Nutritional Medicine	49
On the right track	52
Is Your Doctor Killing You?	53

CHAPTER TWO

WHY ME?	**55**
Types of Cancers	56
Cancer staging	56
Characteristics of Cancer Cells	58
How Cancer Becomes Life-threatening	59
Signs of cancer	60
Avoiding The Risks	61
16 Reasons Why You Get Cancer	62
1. Sunlight	63
2. Chronic exposure to electromagnetic fields (EMFs)	63
3. Ionizing radiation	65
4. Pesticide/herbicide residues	65
5. Industrial toxins	67
6. Polluted, chlorinated and fluoridated water	68
7. Tobacco	68
8. Hormone therapies	69

9. Wrong diet and nutrition 71
10. Emotional stress 73
11. Intestinal toxicity and digestive impairment 73
12. Viruses 74
13. Blocked detoxification pathway 75
14. Cellular oxygen deficiency 75
15. Cellular terrain 76
16. Genetic factors 77
Summary 77

CHAPTER **THREE**

NATURAL MEDICINE **79**
Cancer According To Natural Medicine 81
  Basis of natural medicine 82
  Uses of natural medicine 85
  How natural therapies fight cancer 86
  The natural medicine arsenal 87
Natural Medicine Cocktails 87
  How to design the cocktail 88
  What is the success rate? 89
Three Cancer Strategies 93
  1. Treat cancer using conventional therapy alone 93
  2. Treat cancer using natural therapy alone 93
  3. Combining conventional and natural therapies 94
Design Of A Successful Integrated Program 97
  1. Data collection 97
  2. Selecting the right therapy 97
  3. Selecting the right timing 98
Four Pillars Of A Successful Integrated Cancer Program 98
  1. Emotional and psychological 99
  2. Structural 99
  3. Energy 99
  4. Biochemical 100
Is Natural Medicine for Me? 100
  Step 1. Face reality 101
  Step 2. Do your homework 103
  Step 3. Make the decision 104

CHAPTER **FOUR**

PREVENT MUTATIONS **105**
Free Radicals And Antioxidants 106
Classes Of Antioxidants 107
  Antioxidant enzymes 107
  1. Super oxide dismutase 107
  2. Catalase 108
  3. Glutathion peroxidase 108

Molecular antioxidants 108
 1. Vitamin C 108
 2. Vitamin E 108
 3. Carotenoids 108
 4. Bioflavonoids 109
 5. Minerals 109
Should Antioxidants Be Used? 110
Single Nutrient or Nutritional Cocktail? 114
 Nutrients to avoid 115
Important Cancer Antioxidants 115
 1. Beta-carotene 116
 2. Vitamin C 117
 3. Vitamin E 125
 4. Selenium 126
 5. Lipoic acid 127
 6. Poly-MVA 128
 7. Bioflavonoids 130
  A. Green tea 130
  B. Quecertin 131
  C. Tangeretin 131
  D. Resveratrol 132
What Should You Do? 132

CHAPTER **FIVE**

OPTIMIZING MITOCHONDRIAL FUNCTION **135**
Coenzyme Q10 136
 Human/Clinical studies 137
  Case-study in Denmark 137
  Research study in Texas 138
Magnesium 140
B Complex Vitamins 142

CHAPTER **SIX**

BOOSTING YOUR IMMUNITY **143**
Basics Of The Immune System 144
 1. Cat's Claw 146
 2. Olive Leaf 147
 3. Essiac Herbs 148
 4. Hoxsey Herbs 154
 5. Fish Oil 155
 6. Iscador 157
 7. Medicinal mushroom 158
  A. Maitake mushroom 158
  B. Reishi mushroom 160
  C. Shitake mushroom 162
  D. Agaricus Blazel Murill (ABM) 162

    E. Cordycep sinensis (CS) — 163
  8. Ukrain — 165
  9. Lactoferrin — 166
  10. Inositol Hexaphosphate (IP-6) — 166
Additional Factors to Boost Immunity — 168

CHAPTER **SEVEN**

STOPPING CANCER SPREAD — **169**
How Does Cancer Grow? — 170
Essential Natural Compounds To Stop Cancer Spread — 171
  1. Calcium D-glucarate — 171
  2. Curcumin — 172
  3. Milk thistle — 172
  4. Resveratrol — 173
  5. Powdered shark cartilage — 174
  6. Liquid shark cartilage — 175
  7. Bovine tracheal cartilage (BTC) — 175
  8. Bindweed — 176
  9. Collagen-matrix reinforcement — 177
    A. Vitamin C — 178
    B. L-Lysine — 179
    C. L-Proline — 179
  10. Artemisinin (Wormwood) – from malaria to cancer — 180

CHAPTER **EIGHT**

BALANCED INTERNAL TERRAIN — **187**
Acidity-alkalinity (ph) — 188
  How to test your pH level — 190
    1. Salivary pH test — 190
    2. Urinary pH test — 190
Intestinal Flora — 191
  1. Digestive enzymes — 192
  2. Probiotics — 194
  3. Green foods — 195
  4. Fiber — 197

CHAPTER **NINE**

UNLOAD YOUR TOXINS — **199**
Definition Of Toxins — 201
Types Of Toxins — 201
  1. Toxic metals — 204
  2. Liver toxins — 202
  3. Microbial toxins — 203
  4. Protein by-product toxins — 203
Do We Need Detoxification? — 204
  Benefits of detoxification — 204

Principles Of A Detoxification Program   205
   1. Cleansing   206
     A. Complete fasting   206
     B. Vegetable juicing   206
     C. Skin cleanse   208
     D. Colon cleanse   210
     E. Lung and lymphatic cleanse   212
     F. Kidney and blood cleanse   213
     G. Toxic metal cleanse   214
   2. Rebuilding   206
   3. Maintenance   215
     Cleansing herbal teas   216
The Gerson Therapy Of Detoxification   217

CHAPTER **TEN**

ANTI-CANCER DIET   **219**
Benefits Of A Good Diet   221
Characteristics Of An Anti-cancer Diet   222
   1. Low in sugar   222
   2. High in antioxidants   225
   3. Promoters of an alkaline environment   226
   4. Promoters of the immune system   228
Where Is The Evidence?   228
What Food To Eat?   229
   Dietary principles for easy digestion   231
   Do I have to be a vegetarian?   232
   Whey protein to supplement nutrition   232
How Food-based Antioxidants Fight Cancer   234
Specific Anti-cancer Foods   234
   Carotenoids   235
   Cruciferous vegetables   235
   Laetrile (Amyglalin)   235
   Garlic   236
   Some special considerations   236

CHAPTER **ELEVEN**

OTHER NATURAL THERAPIES   **237**
   Hyperthemia To Kill Cancer Cells   238
   Bioresonance To Induce Cell Decomposition (Lysis)   239
   Ultraviolet Blood Irradiation (Ubi) Therapy   240
   Oxygenating Therapies   240
   Magnetic Therapy   241
   Lymphatic Therapy   242
   Insulin Potentiation Therapy   243
   Zoetron Therapy   243

EPILOG   **245**
REFERENCES   **248**
INDEX   **258**

INTRODUCTION

Over four million Americans are currently under treatment for cancer, with another four million "in remission", awaiting a recurrence of cancer. **The overall 5-year survival rate of many cancers, including liver, lung, pancreas, bone, and advanced breast cancer, has not increased in the past 30 years,** after $45 billion spent on research and seven million casualties. Today, 42% of Americans can expect to develop cancer in his or her lifetime, and 24% are expected to die from it. On a worldwide basis, **cancer is fast replacing heart disease as the number one cause of death in adults.** These are real numbers, and affecting real people, including your loved ones. In fact, the next victim may be you. Effective treatments are lacking for many cancers, especially in advance stages. This book is about how to stay alive if you have cancer. Plain and simple.

This book is written because it's time for conventional doctors to admit that the current medical approach to cancer by cut (surgery), poison (chemotherapy), and burn (radiation therapy) isn't working as well as it should.

The current paradigm started 150 years ago with the advent of drug-based allopathic medicine advocated by Western scientists. What was considered traditional medicine (much of it using natural non-toxic compounds) then, was swept quickly to the side and labeled as quackery. Medical societies set up strict guidelines for physicians to follow, and anyone not abiding by the pre-set protocols had their license revoked, and some were even jailed. For the past century, cancer specialists have been continuing on the same path of treatment which they know are unlikely to make much positive difference in the lives of their patients in the majority of cancer cases. Perhaps this blindness has to do with the sad reality that physicians practicing outside prescribed conventional protocols can and will continue to lose their license, that offending big drug companies that sponsor research can be a big mistake, and being labeled as quacks by their colleagues is no fun. No wonder physicians are afraid of new approaches to healing cancer. **No wonder patients all over the world are moving away from conventional therapies in search of better options.**

The good news is that **more and more doctors are accepting alternative cancer therapy to augment conventional treatment.** I was in the same boat some years back, as a Western-trained allopathic doctor, following the standardized protocol and entrenched policies set down by our respected medical board. It was so much easier then. To learn that there are scientifically sound natural alternatives to cancer therapy is indeed a painful and humbling experience. It is easier to turn away from the truth and continue on the merry way of accepted mediocrity. To face the truth requires that I unlearn many of the "proven" theories of modern medicine, an admission that many such theories taught to us in medical school are downright wrong, and to relearn the real truth of medicine. This requires spending time not with information from drug companies and journals funded by drug companies, but revisiting the biochemistry textbooks, countless hours on Medline to keep up with the latest research, and open discussions with natural-oriented healthcare professionals. In the end, I saw the light. **The light that conventional therapies have failed, that scientifically-based natural non-toxic therapies do exist** and have existed for centuries, and most importantly, should be used in a clinical setting for the benefit of our cancer patients. **We need the best of both worlds, and it is available.**

My message is simple, direct, and lifesaving: **cancer can be beaten using non-toxic natural compounds and modalities in conjunction with conventional therapy. This combination approach is the treatment of choice for most cancers.** This book will show you the logic behind this approach and how to use it. Natural medicine is an effective tool against cancer. It can be beautifully and successfully incorporated into the conventional treatment program in addition to being a stand-alone alternative at times. **There is no "single cure" for cancer and none is proposed,** conventional or otherwise. What is available is the judicious use of multiple natural treatments and natural compounds working together – synergistically – to effect major changes in the cancer process, from containment to remission to a life that is cancer free. In other words, you don't have to become a statistic.

This book is not an attack on the medical profession or conventional treatment protocols which have their place. This book does not promise natural therapy as a sole substitute. This book does advocate the use of natural therapies as an adjunct therapy to most conventional therapies. To do that, we start with exploring the current state of the cancer war and what causes cancer from a natural perspective. Before natural medicine can be taken seriously, its foundational basis must be examined and scrutinized. After we are satisfied with the science behind the concept of natural medicine, we move on to study, one chapter at a time, the parameters within which natural medicine works as an anti-cancer tool. When you have finished the book, I hope that you have a better understanding of our body as it is indeed a miraculous ecosystem and not simply a mechanical device as we were taught to believe; that when the ecosystem is in a dysfunctional state, symptoms such as cancer can arise; most importantly, that this ecosystem can be brought back to homeostasis naturally with non-toxic compounds and lifestyle changes, with resulting reversal of cancer.

As you will see, all of us already have cancer cells in our body, but not all of us will end up with cancer in the hospital. In fact, **the average adult at age 60 will already have about six bouts of cancer without knowing it,** due to the superb job performed by our immune system over the years to keep the cancer in check. When you have a detectable tumor, your goals are clear and specific – how to destroy the trillions of cancer cells that are ravaging your body. The conventional strategy of containment simply does not work due to the sheer number of cancerous cells present and circulating but not detectable by current diagnostic standards. Only by combining traditional strategies of confinement advanced by conventional medicine plus enhancing our body's immune system, together with an optimized internal terrain with natural medicine that is non-toxic, does.

Some of you may think that *"If it were any good, my doctor would know about it".* Yes, your doctor would eventually know. The question is when, and whether you have the time to wait. Dissemination of new information takes decades (likely to be anywhere from 10 to 20 years) and not months in the case of natural medicine.

Much of the scientific information presented here is years ahead of its time. The number of practitioners of natural and nutritional medicine is limited, and those with orthomolecular oncology background even less. I am proud to join my fellow learned colleagues, whose names you may be familiar with, such as cardiologist Robert Atkins, MD, winner of the National Health Federation's Man of the Year Award and author of numerous books including *Dr Atkin's Health Revolution*; Ernesto Contreras MD, chief oncologist at the famed cancer-focused Oasis Hospital in Mexico; conventional and alterative oncologist James Forsythe, MD, HMD, associate professor of medicine at the University of Nevada; and Abram Hoffer, MD, PhD, clinician and author of *Orthomolecular Medicine for Physicians,* to offer patients a balanced approach to cancer treatments. What is proposed in this book isn't the least bit complex or unreasonable. **Natural medicine is the "true" medicine that is time-tested and has been around for centuries. It fact, it is radical only in its common sense approach.** What is proposed, however, is simply outside the current paradigm of conventional medicine, despite the overwhelming science behind many of these therapies.

Now more than ever, we realize that maintaining proper balance is the key to most things in life. Work needs to be balanced with play. Solitude needs to be balanced with social activities. The treatment of choice in most degenerative diseases has now turned from simply reaching a "target" of any single laboratory test "score" to a more complete and balanced approach of managing key ratios. For example, achieving an ideal laboratory total cholesterol level alone is hardly the right strategy to reduce cardiovascular risk. The key is the balance of total cholesterol to HDL cholesterol ratio. Similarly, it is not the total triglyceride in our blood that is a risk factor, rather the total triglyceride to HDL cholesterol ratio. The same applies to the balance of omega-3 to omega-6 fatty acids, estrogen to progesterone and zinc to copper. The list goes on. A balanced approach is indeed needed in cancer treatment. Taking in the best of both conventional and natural medicine in a complementary and integrated fashion makes the most sense if you want to maximize your lifespan, whether you have cancer or not.

If you want to know how to beat cancer with natural medicine, or how to balance the use of natural medicine in the context of conventional therapy to optimize the healing process, this book is for you. If you have cancer but are in remission, you need this book even more as this is precisely the time when natural medicine plays its most profound role, helping to keep the cancer from recurring. If you simply want to know how to prevent cancer naturally, there is no better place to start than here.

As the era of the "kill or cure" approach to conventional cancer therapy draws to a close, the era of natural medicine focusing on biologically supportive therapies is making clear inroads into mainstream oncology. Let us begin the journey of healing.

EXECUTIVE SUMMARY

(Read this section if you don't have time or are too weak to read the whole book.)

WAR ON CANCER

For the past 50 years, war on cancer has been fought with three tools – surgery (cut), radiation therapy (burn), and chemotherapy (poison). Over the same period, there have been rapid improvements in technology and medical science. One would expect medical treatments and success rates for cancer to improve steadily. But have they? The answer is an emphatic no.

Since 1950, the overall cancer incidence has increased by 44%, with breast cancer and male colon cancer up by 60% and prostate cancer up by 100%. **44% of Americans living today are expected to develop cancer.**

For decades, the 5-year survival rate has remained constant for non-localized breast cancer at 18% and lung cancer at 13%. Grouped together, the average cancer patient has a 50/50 chance of living another 5 years, which are the same odds he or she had in 1971.

If one takes a longer view, the numbers become scarier. For example, **the overall 5-year survival rate for breast cancer is about 75%, but the extended survival rate (beyond 5 years) is less then 50%.** For prostate cancer, the picture is not much brighter, with 5-year survival at about 85%, and 10-year survival at only 35%.

CANCER – ACCORDING TO NATURAL MEDICINE

While conventional medicine primarily treats cancer as a focal disease with localized symptoms, naturally oriented physicians think otherwise. Naturally oriented physicians think of the body as a closed internal ecosystem, and believe that it is the dysfunction of this ecosystem that is primarily responsible for the development of cancer.

No treatment, conventional or otherwise, can completely eliminate all cancer cells according to the naturally oriented physician. The reason is simple. **Cancer is a systemic disease,** and there are simply too many cancerous or pro-cancerous cells within the ecosystem of the body. **Cancer is not a localized problem but a whole-body phenomenon of metastatic growth.** Its growth process is affected by biological conditions. Non-genetically based cancer forms in the body because of toxins, the lack of oxygen, poor nutrition, and other factors such as hormonal imbalance. Whether the cancer in our body continues to multiply depends to a large degree on our body's biological terrain. It is this terrain that determines how the cancer is expressed.

Naturally oriented doctors view cancer as a chronic, systemic and metabolic dysfunction of the genetical intracellular makeup. In many cases, it can be considered a **controllable chronic illness.** Tumors are only the symptoms of the submicroscopic dysfunctional causes. The root of cancer therefore lies in the progress of growth and metastasis, and not the tissue in which the tumor was first detected.

The naturally oriented doctor therefore fights cancer by optimizing the internal terrain and enabling the patient's internal system to destroy the tumor. It enhances the patient's health so that cancer cells cannot grow and multiply.

The Rate of Success

The use of non-toxic natural therapies has achieved huge successes over the past few decades. Extensive studies have proven them to have an edge over conventional therapies. Some of the examples are listed below.

Many of the alternative cancer hospitals are found in Mexico. For example, Dr Contreras of the Oasis Hospital reported that his 5-year survival rate for prostate cancer is 83% when using natural treatment compared to 73% for conventional treatment.

At the American Metabolic Institute, renowned scientist Dr Geronimo Rubio reported success rates in reversing stage III and IV cancers from 65 to 75%. The reversal rate for stage I and II cancers is 80%.

While the 5-year survival for ending stage cancer using conventional therapy is 9% overall, alternative cancer hospitals report that theirs is more than 30%. While 4% of terminal cancer patients show no response to alternative treatments, the other 96% can expect some benefits after a month of treatment. There is therefore no turning back for patients who have bravely embarked on the path of alternative treatments.

Clearly, the success rate of natural treatment is so much better than for many conventional cancer treatment. As such, if you or your family members have cancer, you should consider all forms of alternative treatment before deciding on which program to embark on. Today, many patients opt for combination therapy, using both conventional and alternative cancer treatments. This **combined therapy is becoming more and more popular as the success rates are higher.**

Integrating natural and conventional therapies

Human and animal studies have shown successful and amazing results when chemotherapeutic agents and natural compounds are used in combination.

The objectives and rationale behind combining conventional therapies with natural treatments are as follows:

1. To give a safer and more effective dose to reduce the negative side effects.
2. To help build healthy cells' resistance to chemotherapy and radiotherapy and increase drug accumulation in cancer cells.
3. To increase additive or synergistic cytotoxic effect with chemotherapy and radiotherapy.

Know Your Enemy

Here are 10 cancer facts you must know to fight the battle and win.

1. Mitochondria
The mitochondria is the energy factory of the cell. This is the engine room, so to say. **Fortification of mitochondrial function will help cellular energy generation.** Cancer cells prefer sugar as a source of energy as compared to normal cells which favor oxygen. This is an inefficiency pathway of energy generation. This process drains our body of the much-needed energy at a time when the body is weak. As a result, most cancer patients are weak and tired.

2. Free Radicals
Free radicals (very reactive chemical particles) generated as a result of environmental toxins, stress, processed food, and pollution are a direct cause of cellular mutation and cancer. **Blending optimum levels of antioxidants into the therapy is a cornerstone of an anti-cancer program.**

3. Matrix

Cancer cells are commonly harmless or benign. Such benign tumors are encapsulated by fiber and the body is insulated from their toxic effects. Cancer cells spread locally by secreting enzymes that destroy the interstitial collagen that forms the protective intercellular matrix. Reinforcing of this matrix is akin to building a wall and preventing the cancer cells from advancing.

4. Temperature Sensitive

Cancer cells are more sensitive to heat and less able to tolerate high temperature compared to normal cells. Hyperthermia (raising the body temperature) should be induced, including metabolic hyperthermia at the cellular level, to kill cancer cells.

5. Angiogenesis

Cancer cells spread to distant sites by angiogenesis (formation of new blood vessel). Masses of cancer cells may become like parasites, developing their own network of blood vessels and siphoning key nutrients from the body. **Some non-toxic compounds have been shown to retard this process.**

6. Toxins

Many cancers come on because of an excess of toxins and a compromised toxin clearance mechanism in the body. **Detoxification is a key to cancer control.** The liver, skin, kidney, and lung are major detoxification centers of the body.

7. Internal Terrain

Our body is an internal closed ecosystem. The proper balance of this internal terrain by maintaining its equilibrium, for example an optimum acid/base balance, is a key to preventing a buildup of unwanted bacteria, fungus, and proteins (like prions) in the body which can bring on cancer.

8. Immunity

Our first line of defense against assaults by external agents in our body is our immune system. Those who are immunologically strong have a better chance of surviving cancer.

9. Hormones

Most cancers have a hormonal component. The imbalance of our hormones is a major cause of many cancers, including breast and prostate cancer. Modulation and correction of hormonal imbalance naturally will correct the systemic dysfunction upon which hormonal sensitive cancer is kept under control.

10. Inflammation

Infections, poor dietary habit or high sugar and trans-fat are potential carcinogens that leads to mutational changes and an exaggerated inflammatory response that may be out of control resulting in cancer. Side effects of inflammatory response include atherosclerosis, diabetes, stroke, and hypertension.

NATURAL MEDICINE – YOUR CHOICE

Let me help you by outlining the three steps you should take to make this critical decision. No one should embark on a natural medicine program without understanding what it is all about. It is not easy by any means, but has its rewards.

Step 1   Face the reality

Do not deny that you have cancer. All adults do. You just have it more than others. You are not alone, and millions before you have the same. What you have can be beaten.

Do you want to beat cancer? It is being done all the time. Those who have the strongest reason to live also have the best odds of beating cancer. Tell yourself, *"I refuse to die!"* and list out the reasons why. Maybe it is your wish to be with your love ones, or you have a mission still incomplete. Whatever the reasons may be, list them out. Without a reason to fight, no war can be won. Until your reasons for fighting the war on cancer are clear, do not proceed. Take your time to think it through. Talk to your love ones.

Step 2   Do your homework

This is the time to gather as much knowledge, options, and data as possible. It may entail many phone calls, visits to professionals you have never heard of in distant land, exploring options that sounds like foreign language to you. Yes this is uncharted territory for you, and you need to do your homework as quickly as possible. The good news is that there are professionals out there who can help you, and this is the time to call them.

Talk to your doctor; get the official medical diagnosis, the staging, and any variance. Search the Internet for as much information as possible on the cancer you have, from both conventional and alternative sources. Verify that the prognosis and treatment plan advanced by your oncologist conforms to established protocol. Write down on paper questions you may have about your cancer. The more questions the better.

Step 3   Make the decision

After you have gathered all the information, you must make a decision. You only have one body, and you cannot afford not to give it the best.

7 STEPS TO BEATING CANCER NATURALLY

Cancer can be beaten naturally if you are determined.

There are seven things you must do from the natural medicine perspective to control cancer cell growth and beat it. They reflect a complete approach to address the major cancer facts outlined above. **All seven steps are important.** Do not think that one is more important than others. You have to do all if you are serious. Start with step 1, and move on to the next steps, one at a time, while continue to do what the previous step requires. Take your time to conquer each step before moving on. Most people require about three weeks per step. Beating cancer is a marathon and not a sprint. If you can move through the seven steps faster, it is even better.

Step 1 Starving Cancer cell

Cancer is a sugar-feeder. Learn to **cut down the sugar intake** (including granular and refined sugar) **by up to 90%** to create a low sugar environment. You do need food for energy. Change to low-glycemic index complex carbohydrates. Cut off all soda pop, most grains, rice, and potato.

Step 2 Oxygenate your body

Cancer cells hate oxygen. They strive in an anaerobic (oxygen-free) environment. **Moderate aerobic exercise** is the easiest and cheapest way to get oxygen on board. If you are too weak to do exercise, simple deep breathing is a good start. Other oxygen-generating modalities could be considered including ozone and hydrogen peroxide therapy.

Step 3   Avoid Malnutrition

Forty percent of cancer patients die of malnutrition. You need good nutrition, with healthy fats and plant-based proteins to maintain nitrogen balance and muscle strength without aggravating the cancer. The amount of calories you need is determined by your physical activity level. It is easy to get calories in. The challenge is to get nutritious and not empty calories into your body. Stay with **organic whole foods, with plenty of green leafy vegetables, low-glycemic fruits, and beans and legumes for plant-based protein.**

Step 4   Use Nutritional Supplements

Therapeutic nutritional supplement is a cornerstone of the natural medicine because our body simply cannot get enough of them from a regular diet. A blend of at least 30-50 nutrients is needed to:

1. **Prevent mutation** with therapeutic doses of antioxidants.
2. **Enhance mitochondrial function** to increase energy production.
3. **Prevent cancer growth** by blocking its spread.
4. **Enhance immune function** to fight existing cancer cells.

Step 5   Balance Your Internal terrain

Probiotics, enzymes, green food, and fiber are the four key pillars to re-balance your internal milieu and pH. Use these every day to ensure optimum transit time, proper absorption of nutrients from the food you take, and proper balance of good and bad bacteria.

Step 6   Balance Your Toxin Load

Hundreds of toxic chemicals including **mercury, lead, arsenic and cadmium** have accumulated in our body through the years.

Detoxification is a process of cleaning up our ecosystem and giving it a fresh start. The key elements are:

1. **Use pure filtered water** as your only source of liquid, and drink plenty of it. There is no substitute.
2. Enhance our liver function with herbs such as **milk thistle**. Our liver is the main detoxification organ.
3. Use **chelating agents** to bind and remove unwanted metals and minerals.
4. Drink **fresh vegetable juices.** Vegetable juicing floods the body with antioxidants.

Step 7   Balance Your Hormones

Often misunderstood and under-appreciated, hormones have a lot more to do with cancer than we think. This is especially so with hormone-related cancers such as breast, ovary, uterus, and prostate cancers.

Maintaining a balanced hormonal profile naturally is a key to well-being and longevity because we are flooded in the sea of hormones.

OPTIONAL – Explore other natural therapies that are not commonly practiced in conventional medicine, such as hyperthermia, Rife frequency generators, etc. Also not to be forgotten is to actively participate in an on-going support group.

GENERAL CANCER NUTRACEUTICAL MODEL

When it comes to nutrition as a tool to fight cancer, **protocols do not exist.** Each practitioner has, from his or her own experience, arrived at a general model that has worked well.

Here is my general cancer model that serves as a basis for additional components to be added depending on each person's specific requirement. This is not a "protocol", as no such protocol exists when it comes to individualized cancer therapy.

1. Start daily with a good foundational formula consisting of at least the following:

- **Vitamin A** (antioxidant) – 15,000 IU (300% RDA) with no more than 5,000 IU in vitamin A palmitate and the rest in natural mixed beta carotene.
- **Vitamin C** (antioxidant) – 1,000 mg (2,000% RDA)
- **Vitamin E** (antioxidant) – 300 to 400 IU (1,333% RDA) in the form of water dispersible d-alpha tocopherol (the natural form).
- **Selenium** (antioxidant) – 200 mcg (285% RDA) in amino acid complex forms to enhance absorption.
- **Magnesium** (antioxidant) – 300 to 600 mg (125% RDA). The calcium to magnesium ratio should be 1:1.
- **Vitamin B9** (folic acid) – 800 mcg (200% RDA). It is a non-toxic nutrient that protects our chromosomes from mutational damage and cancer.
- **Vitamin B12** – 100 to 1,000 mcg.
- **Chromium** – 200 mcg (166% RDA).
- **Zinc** – 30 mg (200% RDA).
- **Calcium** – 300 to 500 mg (30-50% RDA).
- **Citrus Bioflavonoids** – 100 mg

2. Interstitial matrix and collagen building. This cocktail consists of ascorbic acid and mineral ascobates, L-lysine, L-proline, carnitine, and ascorbyl palmitate and citrus bioflavonoids. Start with 1 gram 3 times a day, working up to 3-4 grams 3 times a day. From 12-20 grams of ascobates, 5 grams of L-lysine, 3 grams of L-proline, and 200-400 mg of ascorbyl palmitate should be the goal. Reduce dosage if diarrhea occurs.

3. Whole food nutritional supplementation to modulate the internal terrain and increase alkalinity. Key nutrients include chlorella, spirulina, green blue algae, wheat grass, and barley grass. 20-40 grams of powered supplementation is required a day.

4. Soluble fiber in your diet to ensure optimum detoxification and smooth bowel movement. At least 15-30 grams of soluble fiber supplementation is needed in addition to a diet rich in raw whole food.

5. The following important anti-cancer nutrients may be required depending on the person:

- Co-enzyme Q10 – 100 to 300 mg.
- Niacinamide – 1,000 to 2,000 mg.
- Vitamin E – 400 to 1,200 IU.
- Fish oil – 3,000 to 5,000 mg.
- Calcium D-glucarate – 200 mg
- Proteolytic digestive enzymes – 2 to 8 tablets three times a day.
- Quercetin – 1,000mg to 3,000 mg.
- Beta carotene – 20,000 to 50,000 IU.
- Green tea extract (decaffeinated) – 200 mg
- Pantothenic acid and pantethine mixed – 500 to 1,000 mg.
- Grape seed extract – 100 to 200 mg.

6. To boost immunity, the following are considered:

- Olive leaf extract – 500 to 2,000 mg.
- Milk thistle extract –150 to 300 mg (80% minimum).
- Tumeric extract – 100 to 200 mg (95% minimum).
- Medical mushroom standardized (maitake, agaricus, and shitake) extracts – 500 mg to 2 grams each.

- Garlic – 500-2,000 mg in concentrated form; equivalent to 1,250 mg garlic bulk or half a clove of fresh garlic.
- Cat's claw extract – 200 to 1500 mg.

7. Essiac Tea (Essence or Brewed)

CONCLUSION

Cancer is not simply localized lumps and bumps that we have been programmed to accept through the years. Cancer in the adult can partly be viewed as a degenerative process with symptoms representative of underlying systemic dysfunction. We all have cancer cells in our bodies. It is only when our body is unable to get rid of the cancer cells that a disease process takes place. This is when we are diagnosed as having the fateful and fearful cancer. What are the underlying system dysfunctions? There are many factors, including emotional stress, diet, drugs and chemicals, infections, genetic mutation and environmental pollutants.

Conventional treatments look at cancer as a disease state. The natural-oriented doctor views cancer as a set of symptoms reflecting underlying disease.

The conventional treatment of surgery, radiation and chemotherapy has been the cornerstone of cancer treatment over the past 50 years. Today, the clinical success of these treatments has reached a ceiling. We need to break through this cure ceiling by trying fresh approaches.

Practitioners of natural therapies range from lay people with no medical training to highly trained doctors who have departed from their mainstream practice. The vast majority are doctors seeking to supplement careful use of conventional therapies with natural approaches and not to replace them.

The complete natural healing program should include a therapeutic blend of vitamins, herbs, minerals and enzymes. Choosing the proper combination and dosage of these natural compounds is an important key to success. This comes with not only experience but also an extensive medical knowledge of the cancer process. It is therefore highly recommended to consult a nutritionally oriented physician with an orthomolecular oncology experience before you start any treatment program.

CHAPTER ONE

MY DOCTOR IS KILLING ME!

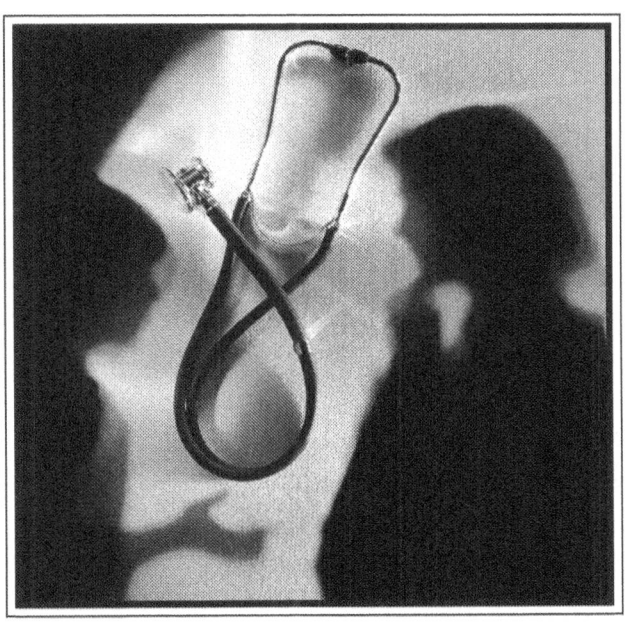

"There is not one,
but many cures for cancer available."

Cardiologist and natural medicine pioneer
Dr Robert Atkins, MD

At the age of 54, Michael Gearin-Tosh was diagnosed in 1995 with myeloma, a bone marrow cancer and one of the most lethal cancers known. Gearin-Tosh is no crackpot. He is a professor in English literature at St. Catherine's College, Oxford, and a visiting professor at Stanford University. His friends include some of the leading conventional oncologists in the world. The usual survival time with conventional treatment is two to three years; without it, one year. Amazingly, seven years later, his cancer is still in remission. Gearin-Tosh remains active and remarkably robust, a fully functioning member of society. The odds against his survival beyond three years were 99.995%. Stories like this are real, and it is happening everyday.

How has he done it? Well, naturally of course. Gearin-Tosh rejected the universally accepted treatment for his form of cancer namely chemotherapy. He fought his cancer with a strong mental determination and a truly remarkable combination of natural therapies, both physical and spiritual. He applied straight diet, detoxification, and a host of natural therapies designed to fortify his body to fight the cancer from within. He consumed enormous daily doses of vitamin C and other antioxidants against the advice of conventional physicians. He did Chinese breathing exercises that date back thousands of years. He did what every conventional doctor advised him against, and he has survived! Gearin-Tosh had a cancer that had been invariably fatal yet he beat it using a combination of exceptionally unconventional natural therapies. In fact, you can read about it in his book, *Living Proof: A Medical Mutiny,* published seven years after his triumph over it.

Gearin-Tosh stayed away from conventional medicine, and that saved his life. Is there a foundation to his madness? Or is his survival just a "lucky coincidence"? Let us explore this more.

Doctors Are the Third Leading Cause of Death In the US!

Seems hard to believe, but the most widely circulated medical periodical in the world, the *Journal of the American Medical Association (JAMA)*, published this information on July 26, 2000.

Studies have shown that **225,000 people die in the US every year because of their doctor.** Sounds incredible! Can it be true? Yes, many have died because of unnecessary surgery (12,000), from wrong prescriptions given (7,000), from hospital infections (80,000), from hospital errors (20,000) and the negative effects of drugs.

In fact, these statistics do not even include the negative effects that are associated with disability or discomfort arising from the above mistakes made.

As if that is not enough, another study, this one published by the same prestigious periodical in 2002, found that **10% of new drugs approved by the Food and Drug Administration (FDA) from 1975 to 1999 have serious side effects that were not discovered during initial testing and marketing.** Dr Karen Lasser and Dr Paul Allen from the Department of Medicine at Cambridge Hospital in Cambridge, Massachusetts found that 56 out of 548 drugs approved during this period (10%) had to have a new "black box warning". When these drugs are consumed, it may have serious adverse reactions that result in death or serious injury. In fact, 16 drugs (3%) were withdrawn and 45 (8.2%) required one or more new black box warnings. Half of the withdrawals occurred during the first two years after the drug's introduction, and half of the new black box warnings occurred during the first seven years. Therefore, **many drugs with adverse effects went undetected until many years later.** One of the drugs, terfenadine (marketed in the US as Seldane) was a popular non-sedating antihistamine. It was on the market for 13 years before it was withdrawn because of arrhythmia.

Another one called cisapride (marketing in the US as Propulsid) was available for six years before it was withdrawn for a similar reason.

Don't these statistics sound scary? We may unknowingly be taking the wrong drugs prescribed by our misguided doctors. We may not realize it now but many years down the road, when the drug is banned, it may have caused irreparable damages to our bodies.

HOW GOOD IS YOUR HEALTHCARE?

Studies have shown that a whopping 20 to 30% of patients in America are receiving inappropriate medical treatment.

Out of 13 countries in a recent comparison of overall health status of its population, the United States ranks an average of 12th, which is second from the bottom for 16 available health indicators. This is indeed not a very good sign. The poor performance of the US health services is also recently confirmed by a World Health Organization survey, which uses different data. Once again, the United States is only number 15 among 25 industrialized countries.

What seems to be the problem? Could this be explained by the lack of medical technology, the lack of qualified doctors, or the lack of financial resources in the United States?

Well, the lack of technology is certainly not a contributing factor to the US's low ranking. Among 29 countries, the United States ranks next to Japan in the availability of highly sophisticated magnetic resonance imaging equipment and computer tomography scanners per million populations. Japan, however, ranks highest while US ranks among the lowest in health services.

The lack of medical education does not seem to be yet another contributing factor. The average American doctor spends about 8 to 10 years in medical training plus additional training in their specialized field. This is much longer as compared to their peers in the rest of the world. The quality and intensity of residency training programs also cannot be questioned. Most of the world's most prestigious medical schools and research facilities are in America.

The US is definitely not lacking in financial resources. The US is rich and the amount of money spent on healthcare ranks among the top in the world.

A real problem therefore exists in the entire allopathic medical system of healthcare and philosophy characteristic of Western medicine. Western trained doctors are highly focused on alleviation of symptoms and eradication of localized problem. They fail miserably when it comes to eliminating the underlying systemic problem that is often the root of the many age-related degenerative diseases such as hypertension, diabetes, atherosclerosis, and cancer. The failure to accept cancer as a systemic disease is one of the greatest failures in modern medicine.

In the words of Vincent Speckhart, MD, MDH, renowned practicing oncologist of 22 years' experience:

*Cancer growth is looked upon as a problem and a disease, when in fact it is the result of failure of the host in which it is growing to maintain a healed state.****Treating cancer as a disease state without attention to the underlying cause is a grave mistake.***

– Vincent Speckhart, past assistant clinical professor of medicine at Eastern Virginia Medical College. Homeopath since 1989.

If cancer is a localized problem, the traditional model will serve well. The reality is very different. **Cancer is really a systemic disease with local manifestation.** Until the root of the systemic dysfunction is eradicated, symptomatic treatments and local eradication is a band-aid temporary approach at best. The fact speaks for itself. For the past half a century, the three accepted modalities of treatment – surgery, chemotherapy, and radiation therapy – has remained essentially unchanged in conceptual terms. There has been no significant breakthrough.

On the other hand, the number of Americans diagnosed annually with cancer will double over the next 50 years, from 1.3 million to 2.6 million. Researchers estimated that 8.9 million people were living with cancer in the United States at the beginning of 1999. About 60% of those were 65 or older. As the population continues to age, the incidence of cancer and the need for breakthrough rises. By 2050, more than 1.1 million people 75 and older will be diagnosed with the disease each year, up from about 400,000 today, according to a study released by the National Cancer Institute.

Such being the case, little wonder more and more cancer patients no longer opt for traditional therapies as the only option to treating their cancer. The conventional methods do not seem to work and in some cases, they have even shortened the patients' lives. Conventional allopathic doctors simply have nothing better to offer. Many patients have lost faith in them. Once bitten, twice shy, many cancer patients now look for alternative therapies.

Statistics show that **40 to 80% of cancer patients are seeking alternative cancer treatments either in conjunction with or in place of conventional treatment.**

ADULT CANCER – A DEGENERATIVE DISEASE?

Statisticians further tell us that 80% of us will die from heart disease, stroke and/or cancer one day. The World Health Organization has estimated that there will be more than ten million documented new cases of cancer a year. In fact, cancer is fast replacing cardiovascular disease as the number one cause of death among adults.

We all know that heart disease and stroke are old people's diseases. Children very seldom get heart attacks or strokes. But cancer can happen to all of us, whether you are a grandparent or an active pre-school child. Long ago, during the times of our great grandparents, cancer was looked upon as a form of sickness and a "curse" that just appeared and that was not related to the aging process. Therefore, when we get it, we get it. There is really nothing we can do about it. Let us take a closer look at this hypothesis. The incidence of adult cancers hit a peak around age 50. The lowest incidence of adult cancer is between ages 30 to 35. Why? Let us consider the aging process first.

When we are around the age of 20 to 25 years old, our body reaches its peak of condition, that is, our health is likely to be at its highest point. Our hormone production will start to decelerate and we gradually begin our journey of aging. We enter into the Sub-clinical Phase of aging at age 25 as our cellular function begins its gradual decline, although it seems unnoticeable. At this point in time, we may still feel very youthful. The thought of growing old is definitely far away from our minds and there is no outward sign of any deterioration. This phase goes on from age 25 to 35.

As we grow older, say between age 35 to 45, the so-called Transition Phase of aging, symptoms such as a lower energy level and wrinkles will be noticed. We may start to have hypothyroidism, resulting from the decline of thyroid hormone levels. We may also start to feel more lethargic and tired because of the decline in growth hormones. This is when some dreaded diseases such as diabetes may set in due to the onset of insulin and sugar imbalance. The incidence of cancer is still small at this stage compared to hypertension, diabetes, and atherosclerosis.

Age 45 and above is the age of prosperity. Not only do we prosper in our career, we also prosper in old age diseases! We have now entered the Clinical Phase of aging. Signs and symptoms of aging become very obvious. Many of us can no longer hide our age. Our hormone levels start to decline rapidly. We may reach our next milestone of menopause and andropause. Cancer, hypertension, and heart attacks are feared universally as they strike two out of three adults at this age. Cancer has now become one of the most common diseases of all adults in this group.

Why does cancer hit most frequently when we are in our 50s and not in our 30s? The answer is simple. At age 50, we are older, and our body is weaker. It's common sense. Extending this hypothesis, is it not true that the longer we can stay young, the less likely it is that cancer will surface? Very few can argue against this, and the simplicity of this statement points to the very essence of **adult cancer – that it is primarily an age-related disease.**

Let us take a look at what the aging process does to your body to excite cancer cells. Our healthy bodies are in a continuous state of balance and homeostasis. When we are physically or emotionally stressed, imbalances will occur. The body will automatically adjust and try to re-balance itself. If this compensatory mechanism fails, we fall sick with outward symptoms such as pain or fever.

Sometimes, we are sick inside without any outward symptoms because the body is able to compensate for the dysfunction without us knowing it. Due to the lack of sophisticated detection equipment, we may not know that we already have some disease such as hypertension, diabetes and cancer. In reality, they may already be well into their **"sub-clinical" state** and affecting various parts of our bodily function. Hypertension is often called the "silent killer", and for a good reason. It may kill you before you know it. Cancer is another one.

As medical science progresses, we will be able to design sophisticated tests to detect such dysfunction earlier. We now have total body CT scans, and well advanced cardiac markers such as homocysteine and lipoprotein(a) to help us screen potential cardiac problems ahead of time.

In the case of cancer, no one standardized and universally accepted screening measurement has yet been developed. Tumor markers as a screening tool are not very reliable and most of them are relatively crude. Until the cancer presents itself as a growth or show up on a scan, the patients are considered "normal". Most people are surprised when they learn that they have cancer. Why? Because they never thought that they would be the one afflicted since there never was any sign of it. Ironically, the first symptom of cancer, according to a patient education brochure published by the American Cancer Society is "no symptom". In a world dominated by allopathic medicine where the focus of treatment is on symptomatic relief, how can a doctor treat cancer where there are no symptoms? And how can a patient prevent cancer when there are no indicators to warrant prevention in the first place?

In reality, **all of us are born with pre-cancerous cells.** Louis Pasteur, the famous Frenchman who brought us the germ theory of disease, is a name we all recognize. The milk we take is "pasteurized" to rid it of unwanted bacteria which he proved to be the cause of disease. A body in its pristine state, therefore, will not get sick, according to the thinking of that time more than a century ago. We now know that this is incorrect, for a pristine body simply does not exist. Pasteur, on his death bed in 1895, admitted as much and said, *"I have been wrong. The germ is nothing. The 'terrain' is everything".*

What exactly is this terrain that Pasteur alluded to? The terrain is our internal ecosystem. It is a closed system that works 24 hours a day to keep us going. It is made up of 65 trillion cells modulated by acid/base balance, hormonal influences, structural functionality, and a delicate balance between good and bad bacteria already present from birth. It is the dysfunction of this internal terrain that accounts for most of our diseases, including cancer.

"What disrupts our internal terrain?" you may ask. The key elements are diet, lifestyle, stress, and environmental pollution, not to mention genetic factors. These insults come on slowly and insidiously.

We now know that 80 to 90% of all cancers are related to three major groups of risk factors:

1. **Nutrition** – a high-fat, high-cholesterol, low-fiber, high-sugar diet.
2. **Lifestyle** – alcohol, smoking, stress, sedentary lifestyle.
3. **Environment** – industrial toxics, electromagnetic radiation, chemical carcinogens, air and water pollution, among others.

Our body is constantly being attacked when exposed to these risk factors. Unfortunately, the insults are so small that they are not noticed, and it takes on average 20 years or more before symptoms of the first damage become outwardly evident. These insults attack our cellular protein structure, causing mutational changes that can lead to cancer and a variety of chronic degenerative diseases, including hypertension and diabetes. **By the age of 50, it is**

estimated that 30% of our cellular proteins will have been damaged. Is there any surprise that this is the time cancer surfaces most frequently?

It is, therefore, fair to say that all adults (and some children) have cancerous cells in their bodies. These cells exist in a sub-clinical state, suppressed by our internal immunity system in their quest to keep our internal ecosystem or internal terrain functioning optimally. When these attacks are chronic, that is when they are sustained over time, our defense system will eventually fail, and the sub-clinical state of dysfunction will manifest itself with physical symptoms. The symptoms include lumps which contain cancerous cells. This illustrates cancer as a process of abnormal cellular growth caused by an underlying dysfunctional state of the body's internal terrain in the majority of cases. Cancer is simply not a lump or mass that "just comes on" without any reason.

Julian Whitaker, MD, noted alternative cancer expert, sums up his view of cancer this way:

I look upon cancer in the same way that I look upon heart disease, arthritis, high blood pressure, or even obesity, for that matter, in that by dramatically strengthening the body's immune system through diet, nutritional supplements, and exercise, the body can rid itself of the cancer, just as it does in other degenerative diseases. Consequently, I wouldn't have chemotherapy and radiation because I'm not interested in therapies that cripple the immune system, and, in my opinion, virtually ensure failure for the majority of cancer patients.

Although advance technology and science have stretched man's life expectancy from 42 to 76 years over the last century, more and more people are still getting cancer. In fact, one in three adults will die of cancer. The lifetime chance of getting cancer of the colon is

6%, the prostate 17%, the breast 14%, and the lung 7%. There is evidence that we can reduce the incidence of cancer of the colon by up to 50%, the prostate by 15% and the lung by 90%. That means, we can actually reduce our probability of getting cancer if we really want to!

The good news is that cancer is no longer the death warrant it used to be if you detect and heal it early. Like other diseases such as heart disease and diabetes, the majority of cancers that afflict adults can be viewed as an age-related degenerative disease in conceptual terms. This will help us understand the many facets of cancer pathology and why it can be overcome naturally, just like diabetes and atherosclerosis. Today, advance medical science and technology have made it possible for many of these chronic degenerative diseases to be cured if treatment begins early with the correct and appropriate approach.

CONVENTIONAL THERAPIES – HITTING A PLATEAU

Over the past half a century, there have been rapid improvements in technology and medical science. One would expect medical treatments and success rates for cancer to improve steadily. But have they? The answer is an emphatic no. Since 1950, the overall cancer incidence has increased by 44%, with breast cancer and male colon cancer up by 60% and prostate cancer up by 100%. 44% of Americans living today are expected to develop cancer. For decades, the 5-year survival rate has remained constant for non-localized breast cancer at 18% and lung cancer at 13%. Grouped together, the average cancer patient has a 50/50 chance of living another five years, which are the same odds he or she had in 1971.

Depending on which expert you talk to, the war on cancer declared by President Richard Nixon on Dec 23, 1971 has at best been "progressing slowly", and at worse, a "dismal failure" considering the 45 billion dollars spent over the past few decades on cancer research. While the National Cancer Institute (NCI) claims that the 5-year survival rate (the accepted definition of a "cure") has increased from 20% of cancer patients in 1930 to 53% of adults and 70% of children today, critics of the NCI claim that living five years after cancer diagnosis has more to do with earlier diagnosis alone than the therapeutic modalities used.

Let us first take a look on the three accepted conventional cancer treatments – surgery, chemotherapy or radiation therapy.

Surgery (Cut)

Surgery is the most successful conventional treatment. It is very effective in removing localized tumors. If the cancer has spread to other parts of the body, it is far less successful. Debulking by surgical means is also very effective in treating life-threatening and advance-stage cancers.

So we see that surgery can be a useful therapy in some cancers. However, it is seldom necessary in prostate cancer. In breast cancer, a good surgical excision can cure it when combined with non-toxic natural therapies together with detoxification and/or drugs.

Chemotherapy (Poison)

Drugs used in chemotherapy were derived from mustard gas experiments during World War I and II. There is no doubt that cancer cells are easily destroyed during chemotherapy. Unfortunately, cancer cells rely on processes that are similar to those used by normal cells. The difference between cancer cells and normal cells lies in their activities and not in their functions. Hence, chemotherapy gives rise to complications as normal cells that exist alongside the cancer tissues are also damaged during the process.

Another negative side effect is that many chemotherapy drugs have mutagenic properties that cause abnormal changes in DNA. If the patient is pregnant, it may affect the fetus or embryo, leading to birth defects. Some drugs also cause localized skin irritations. It is a sad fact that many patients often die from these side effects or from the drugs themselves due to their high toxicity.

In a survey conducted, 73% of doctors said they would never opt for chemotherapy due to its high toxicity and ineffectiveness if they were inflicted with cancer. This alone tells you how toxic chemotherapy is.

Chemotherapy is so dangerously toxic that it is best avoided in the treatment of most types of cancers. It should only be used when it is proven to be effective and curative, such as for testicular cancer, many children's tumor, and extreme cases of Hodgkin's lymphoma.

Bear in mind that despite the extensive damage done to the body, **chemotherapy can only benefit a small number of epithelial cell cancers** such as cancer of the breast, lungs, prostate, and colon. It can eradicate only about 7% of all human cancers. It looks like opting for chemotherapy may give a cancer patient more liabilities than assets.

In some cases, chemotherapy can perhaps prolong life for another 15% of patients, after which the natural progression of the disease will lead to death. Statistics show that **chemotherapy is not very effective in the treatment of about 80% of malignant tumors.** This is very discouraging. There is a need to climb beyond the current cure plateau by trying new approaches.

If the proven success rates of chemotherapy are so poor, then why do so many people still opt for it? The reason is due to the lack of alternative approaches that are approved by the FDA (Food and Drug Administration). The FDA is supposed to be the watchdog of our nations' health. Unfortunately, when it comes to alternative cancer therapy, it is years behind other countries in Western Europe. Much of this has to do with the politics of cancer and its beneficiary, the pharmaceutical industry.

This is a quote from Ralph Moss, PhD, author of *The Cancer Industry* which perhaps sums up the situation succinctly:

If you can shrink the tumor 50% or more for 28 days you have got the FDA's definition of an active drug. That is called a response rate, so you have a response...(but) when you look to see if there is any life prolongation from taking this treatment what you find is all kinds of hocus pocus and song and dance about the disease free survival, and this and that. In the end there is no proof that chemotherapy in the vast majority of cases actually extends life, and this is the GREAT LIE about chemotherapy, that somehow there is a correlation between shrinking a tumor and extending the life of the patient.

The inescapable fact is that chemotherapeutic agents are toxic and can cause a great deal of collateral damage to the body. It lowers the person's natural resistance to diseases as it suppresses the immune system. In addition, the toxic nature of the treatment is feared almost as much as the cancer itself. Whether the patient survives long after that is a gamble.

In a research study by Dr Ulrich Abel, he concluded that strong and aggressive chemotherapy actually shortens the lives of cancer patients when compared with patients where chemotherapy is either delayed or administered in a lower dosage. He also noted that the temporary shrinking of a tumor growth may not be necessarily a good sign as the remaining cancer cells often become more resistant and multiply more quickly.

Radiation Therapy (Burn)

The final option, radiation treatment, has similar side effects as chemotherapy. The radiation's effective use in palliative treatment for selected cancers cannot be doubted, but generally speaking, **radiation treatment should only be administered very selectively.** In the case of breast cancer, for example, radiation treatment has been shown to reduce death by 13.2%. However, the increase in deaths from other causes, mostly heart disease, goes up by 21.2%. In other words, "The treatment was a success but the patient died".

Although radiation therapy is less painful, people very seldom choose this as the first line of defense because of the unknowns. It is chosen primarily in later-stage cancers where it is used to shrink the tumors encroaching or impinging on vital parts of the body.

Another drawback about this therapy is that there is a certain limit to the radiation that a patient can tolerate. Once a person has been exposed to that lifetime limit, that's it. They cannot take any more beyond this limit. Otherwise, they may die from radiation poisoning. Thus, the exposure to radiation is said to have a cumulative effect.

So is today's conventional cancer treatment of surgery, chemotherapy and radiological therapy the ideal solution? The answer must be "no".

Side Effects

The list of side effects that accompany conventional cancer treatment is indeed scary. They include:

- Bone marrow suppression
- Reactivation of viral diseases such as herpes
- Weakness

- Kidney damage
- Peripheral nerve injury
- Anemia
- Heart muscle damage
- Toxic overload
- Diarrhea
- Hair loss

Worse yet, the success rate, as alluded to above, has remained the same in 30 years. Clearly, something is wrong with conventional therapy. The foundational philosophy of allopathic medical system is that most diseases have a single and definable causative enemy that can be surgically removed or blasted into submission with chemo- and radiation therapy. In a small number of cases, this has been proven correct. In the vast majority of cancers, however, the three tools we have developed are simply not enough to eradicate cancer cells.

We have spent more than half a century focusing all our energies on these three areas and ridiculed any new ideas, and the results speak for themselves. No wonder patients are disillusioned with the current system. Statistics show that over 40% of all cancer patients are seeking alternative treatments, and for good reasons. They are taking their health into their own hands because they have lost faith in their doctor.

A cancer toolbox containing only three tools is far from complete. We need a toolbox with hundreds of tools we can pick and choose from to get the job done. The tools of chemotherapy, surgery, and radiation are simply insufficient. There are many alternative cancer therapies that are valuable assets in cancer treatment. There is no "magic bullet", and none should be expected. What are available, however, are sound natural non-toxic therapies that have been around for centuries but that have been suppressed and ignored by the medical community for the past 100 years. It's time we take a second look at these natural therapies.

WAR ON CANCER – WHO IS WINNING?

Given the limited tools we have to fight cancer, is there any surprise that we are losing the war on cancer? If you are still not convinced that the battle was lost long ago, here are some more facts you should know.

From 1973 to 1987, melanoma increased by 83%, non-Hodgkin's lymphoma by 51%, lung cancer by 32%. The 30-year trend (1960-62 to 1990-92) for death from lung cancer is up 85% for men and up 438% for women, up 29% for prostate cancer, up 4% for breast cancer, up 12% for female pancreatic cancer. The rate of death from some cancers has dropped over the same period: colon and rectum cancers, -9%, male leukemia, -9%, and cancer of the ovary, -8%. Overall, the cancer death rate, after adjusting for changes in the size and composition of the population with respect to age, went up by 7% between 1975 and 1990. Clearly, conventional medicine has failed in its "war on cancer".

Spokesman for conventional care frequently cite the 5-year survival rate as indicative of progress and money wisely spent. In reality, this number is very misleading as can be seen upon close scrutiny.

Between 1974-76 and 1981-87, the 5-year survival rates only rose 2%, from 49% to 51% overall. For cancers of the liver, lung, pancreas, bone, and breast, 5-year survival rates are about the same as they were in 1965. **Due to advances in diagnostic modalities, survival time is now longer than in the past but this is more because of earlier diagnosis than more successful treatment.** For example, consider a woman whose breast cancer is diagnosed three years earlier because of mammography. This woman may live for seven years. In 1985, using older diagnostic and treatment tools, this same woman would have appeared to live only four years. The sad reality is that we have improved on screening tools, but not curing tools. The perceived "success" has only occurred on paper.

Let us look at some additional hard statistics on common cancers. The approximate 5-year survival rate (all stages) using conventional treatment for bladder cancer is 80.7%, 75% for breast cancer, 61% for colorectal cancer, 57% for kidney cancer, 68% for leukemia, 13% for lung cancer, 86% for melanoma, 51% for non-Hodgkin's lymphoma, 44% for ovarian cancer, 3.6% for pancreatic cancer, 85% for prostate cancer, and 68% for uterine cancer. Based on these you may feel pretty good, assuming that after five years, your chances of survival are the same based on a straight-line projection going forward.

If one takes a longer view, the numbers become scarier. For example, the overall 5-year survival rate for breast cancer is about 75%, but the extended survival rate (beyond 5 years) is less then 50%. For prostate cancer, the picture is not much brighter, with 10-year survival only around 35%. A 5-year window and definition of "cure" is not long enough. With the aging population, a 10-year time frame is more appropriate.

Was there cancer on the face of this world before the advent of modern medicine? Of course there was. How did people treat cancer for the past 5,000 years of human history? Did they simply lay there and die? Of course not. Through the centuries, natural therapies were available and had been used by emperors and kings alike to combat cancer. Unfortunately, their use have all but been suppressed the past century and labeled "quackery" by modern medicine. Here is what a respected alternative cancer specialist has to say:

We know that conventional therapy doesn't work – if it did, you would not fear cancer any more than you fear

pneumonia. *It is the utter lack of certainty as to the outcome of conventional treatment that virtually screams for more freedom of choice in the area of cancer therapy. Yet most so-called alternative therapies regardless of potential or proven benefit, are outlawed, which forces patients to submit to the failures we know don't work, because there is no other choice.*

...I'd turn my back on 50 years of institutionalized expertise, because it follows the wrong paradigm. Everything that is done in medicine today or in any other discipline fits some paradigm. The paradigm I use for cancer is that it is a systemic problem in which the normal control mechanisms of your body are altered. Your immune system likely bears the largest burden for this control; thus, all techniques that enhance it are promising. Those that damage it are not.

— Julian Whitaker, MD

NATURAL VS. CONVENTIONAL MEDICINE

The power of natural medicine or therapies to treat cancer has been used for centuries by millions, much longer than drugs which only came on the scene some 150 years ago. Its use had often been underestimated. Today, we know that many of these natural compounds are truly amazing fellows – they are of different structures, sizes, colors and tastes but each contains a nutrition nugget with specific anti-cancer properties.

Most natural compounds used for treating cancer are relatively non-toxic. From laboratory test, we know that their toxicity ranges from 21- to 270-fold less toxic when compared with toxic chemotherapy drugs. Side effects are much less and usually have to do with discomfort, if any, rather than potentially life-threatening outcomes.

Conventional therapy attempts to remove the tumor in cancer patients as much as possible. These highly toxic treatments are of course necessary and life saving at times. But, the bad thing is that they weaken the patient, depleting the body's nutritional reserves and destroying the patient's immunity system at a time when it is needed most. **Natural compounds, on the other hand, boost the body's immunity so that it can fight the cancerous cells.** Cancer cells need to be attacked from many levels. **A shotgun approach is needed,** as we have yet to develop the magic bullet. In addition to focusing on the local lesion with conventional therapy, the comprehensive cancer program needs to consider adjustment of the dysfunctional internal terrain as an integral part of the treatment plan. This is where natural therapies come into play.

Natural therapies are what will be discussed further in this book. Combining the best of drug based and natural based medicine represents the best one-two punch to beat cancer.

NUTRITIONAL MEDICINE

Food-based nutritional supplementation prescribed by natural medicine physicians to cure disease is as old as the history of mankind itself. As a medical sub-specialty within the system of medicine, its advent was made possible only in the mid-1980s. Prior to that, we simply did not have the sophisticated technology to accurately measure, at the cellular level, the impact of natural substances and their effects. The modern era of life sciences, stem cell and genetic research brings with it tools that allow researchers today to measure the amount of oxidative stress, free radical pathology, genetic damage, and mitochondrial function of the cell previously not possible. This is a new science of cellular medicine that was born out of technology.

The basis of natural medicine is the use of food-based nutrition and other non-toxic natural compounds and modalities to optimize cellular function. They correct dysfunctional cellular states such as mutational changes characteristic of cancer.

Unfortunately, most doctors are seldom taught about nutrition during their long medical training to make them comfortable with the use of nutrition as a therapeutic tool. Jean Mayer, a well-known nutritionist, made this humorous comment, *"Do you know that the **average doctor knows only a little more about nutrition than the average secretary? If the secretary has a weight problem, she will probably know more than the average doctor!"***

Out of the 125 medical schools in the United States, only a small percentage require coursework in nutrition. Furthermore, this coursework only comprises just a few hours of lectures on nutrition during their entire training. This is definitely not enough to cultivate a thorough understanding of the relationship between nutrition and health and certainly not enough to qualify the average physician as an expert in this field.

The topic of nutrition is very important in the diagnosis and treatment of many sub-clinical disease states including cancer. But due to the doctor's lack of education and understanding on this topic, they often do not include this as an effective method of treating and preventing diseases. The use of nutrition as a therapeutic tool in the cancer setting is called orthomolecular oncology. A complete cancer treatment program should include such a component. The reason is simple: **40% of cancer patients do not die from cancer itself. They die from malnutrition. Also 67% cancer patients die from a severely depressed immunity system often resulting from aggressive chemotherapy treatments.** In both cases, **death can actually be prevented or delayed with optimum nutritional balance.**

If only these doctors are better versed in nutrition, more lives can be saved. Till today, believe it or not, many of the top doctors know little about nutrition. How can this be true? Well, here are some of the reasons:

1. They have not been taught nutrition in medical school. They are discouraged from practicing this in the clinical setting as it is classified as non-traditional.
2. They do not have the time. They are too busy in their practice to keep abreast with the latest developments in nutritional and natural medicine.
3. They do not have control over the kind of treatment offered to patients. Very often, insurance companies dictate to them. Doctors have to prescribe from a list of approved medication. Natural medicine and herbal remedies are not included in this list.
4. Doctors are afraid to stand out from their peers and be criticized. They usually follow their guidelines strictly.
5. Doctors are generally not flexible. They are conservative and resistant to new changes.

It is wrong to assert that mainstream medicine and conventional cancer therapies are out of fashion and not effective altogether. There is no doubt that these traditional methods can save lives at times. Highly trained doctors have been able to manage acute illness through these conventional methods and they have done well in treating the patients. On this note, proper credit should be given.

To look at it in a different light, you cannot blame your doctor for not offering you alternative therapies either. Chances are not only does he lack the knowledge, but he is also bound by strict medical society rules to stick to conventional protocols. Failure to do so constitutes sub-standard care and even malpractice. Do you then expect your doctor to sacrifice his whole life and career for your sake? Like you, he is the victim of the circumstances.

The issue is certainly complex, and according to Samuel Epstein, MD, "We are not dealing with a scientific problem. We are dealing with a political issue."

ON THE RIGHT TRACK

To successfully treat cancer patients, your doctor must be a generalist and examine in detail the underlying factors that cause the cancer. He must understand fully not only the physiology of the symptoms, but also look into the nutrition and diet, the physical and emotional well-being of the patient. The doctor therefore should be well versed in conventional treatment options as well as scientifically based natural modalities.

To successfully overcome cancer, the patient must understand that he is embarking on an **intensive healing process to reverse or slow down a condition that has accumulated from many years of toxic buildup and dysfunction.** Those who embark on the program early have better chances of recovery.

To successfully chart out a cancer treatment protocol, the patient and doctor must work together to integrate both conventional and natural therapies.

We quote here some reassuring words:

The combination of nutritional therapy plus standard approach is a highly promising comprehensive approach to cancer treatment. Patients who follow this combined approach for at least 2 months have a significantly better outcome than patients on standard therapy alone.

—Abram Hoffer, MD, PhD, author of over 500 medical articles, and nine books, including *Smart Nutrients*, *Vitamin C and Cancer,* and *Orthomolecular Medicine for Physicians,* and an alternative cancer physician of over 770 patients.

IS YOUR DOCTOR KILLING YOU?

Doctors are trained as humanitarians. There is no intention to commit any harm of course. They spend years in training for the purpose of saving lives the best that they can. In the case of cancer therapy, however, their best is simply not good enough because the treatment forms have been misguided.

The fact is that millions of innocent cancer patients have died under the watchful eyes of conventional cancer therapy in the past 30 years. Surely not all of these deaths can be prevented by any medicine, conventional or otherwise. At the same time, there is little doubt that many lives have been lost prematurely from conventional medicine's approach of cut, burn, and poison.

The title of this chapter probably represents the thinking of most cancer patients who have chosen the path of natural therapy, and the conviction of many of those who have suffered unnecessarily because of conventional cancer therapy. Nevertheless, we must make it clear that No, your doctor is not killing you, at least not on purpose! But Yes, you have options, and these options are often not disclosed to you. I also believe that you have a right to know about ALL the options, for it is your body. You are making life and death decisions, and your information must be complete. Only you can decide the proper treatment program, and you can only make an informed decision after you have all the facts, not part of the facts, or only the facts that doctors like you to know.

The good news is that more and more doctors now have an open mind and are starting to offer natural non-toxic therapies to cancer patients as adjunct treatment options to complement their conventional protocols. We are indeed embarking on a new era of healing, combining the best of conventional and natural therapy in our quest to beat cancer.

Now let us learn what cancer is from the latest break-through in science, and how natural medicine fits into the picture.

CHAPTER TWO

WHY ME?

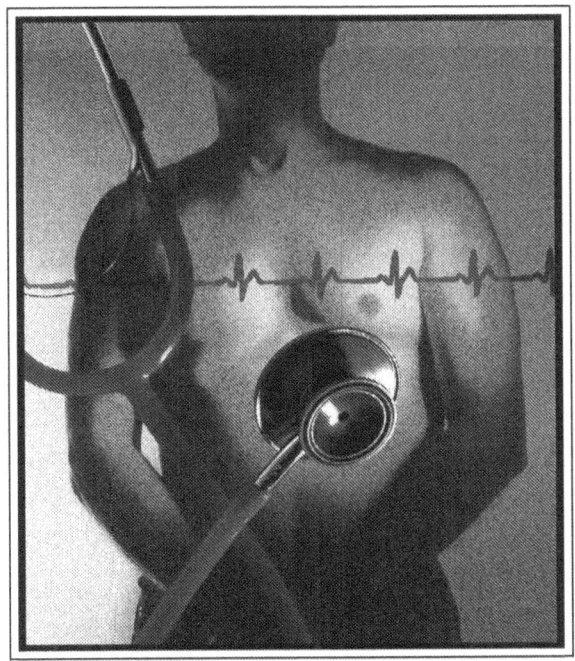

"The important thing is not to stop questioning.
Curiosity has its own reason for existing."

Albert Einstein

B elieve it or not, we know a lot more about why we get cancer than you think. Only by knowing the reasons can we start to beat it. If you have cancer, or know someone who has, this chapter will help you identify some of the risk factors, or even pinpoint the reasons why cancer attacks some while sparing others. Before we do that, let us make sure we are speaking the same language and have a common reference point.

TYPES OF CANCERS

According to conventional allopathic medicine there are over 150 types of cancers that can be categorized as follows:

1. Lung, breast, prostate, skin, stomach, and colon cancers are called carcinomas and are characterized by solid tumors.
2. Sarcomas are cancers that form in the bone and the soft tissues surrounding organs. They are solids and are the most rare and deadly forms of malignant tumors.
3. Leukemia forms in the blood and the bone marrow. These are non-solid tumors and are characterized by abnormal production of white blood cells.
4. Lymphomas are cancers of the lymph nodes. They are divided into two categories, Hodgkin's and Non-Hodgkin's.
5. Myelomas are rare tumors that form in the antibodies producing plasma cells in various tissues.

Cancer Staging

Depending on the type of cancer and the severity of it on diagnosis, conventional treatment options will vary according to how advance the cancer process is. Fortunately, conventional doctors have devised a "staging" system for each cancer for easy reference. All physicians, natural or conventional, need this common reference system before they can start helping you. If you have cancer, it is of paramount importance that you ask your conventional doctor the following:

- **The Medical Name of Your Cancer.** You will need the full medical name in order to research accurately the cancer.

- **The Stage of Your Cancer.** This describes how far cancer has spread. It is usually from stage I to IV, and often followed by "A" or "B" to further delineate the severity within each stage. In general, stage I cancers are small localized cancers that are usually curable, while stage IV usually represents inoperable or metastatic cancer. Stage II and III cancers are usually locally advanced and/or with involvement of local lymph nodes. It is important to note that the staging system is different for each kind of cancer. For solid tumors, stages I-IV are actually defined in terms of a more detailed staging system called the "TNM" system. In the TNM system, TNM stands for Tumor, Nodes, and Metastases. Each of these is separately classified with a number to give the total stage. For example, a T2N1M0 cancer means the patient has a T2 tumor, N1 lymph node involvement, and no distant metastases. Again, the definitions of T, N and M are specific to each cancer.

- **Possibly the Grade of Your Cancer.** Tumor grade refers to a measure of how abnormal the cells in your tumor are when examined under the microscope. This can refer to the appearance of the cells or to the percentage of cancer cells that appear to be dividing abnormally. The higher the grade, the more aggressive and fast growing and devastating the cancer. Tumors are typically classified from least to most aggressive as grade I through IV.

- **Possibly Other Prognostic Factors.** Often, there are specific molecular tests on your cancer cells that may play a significant role in determining treatment and prognosis. For example, breast cancer can be found to be Estrogen Receptor Positive (ER+) or Negative (ER-). ER+ cells have receptors for estrogen on their surface, and their growth often requires the presence of estrogen. ER+ tumors are more affected by hormonal treatment and tend to be less aggressive.

Characteristics of Cancer Cells

After the billions spent on research, we now know the following characteristics of cancer cells. These characteristics are of fundamental importance. All cancer treatments, conventional or otherwise, focus on manipulating the cell and its environment. Knowing the characteristics is therefore a key to winning the cancer war.

These characteristics are:

- Cancer cells have greatly prolonged life spans compared to normal cells.
- Cancer cells fail to develop the specialized functions of their normal counterparts.
- Masses of cancer cells may become like parasites, developing their own network of blood vessels and siphoning off key nutrients from the body.
- Cancer cells prefer sugar as source of energy as compared to normal cells which favor oxygen.
- Cancer cells are more sensitive to heat and less able to tolerate high temperature compared to normal cells.
- Cancer cells form a tumor, or a swelling caused by the abnormal growth if left unchecked. The tumor can invade adjacent normal tissue or spread through lymph vessels or the blood vessels to other normal tissues.

- Cancer cells are usually benign and are carried by many people within their body. Such benign tumors are encapsulated by fiber and insulated from the body and from their toxins.
- Cancers that metastasize quickly are less mature and more aggressive. They are more malignant. An aggressive cancer has a doubling time of 60 days or less; a moderate cancer doubles in 61-150 days, and a indolent cancer doubles in 151-300 days, and a very indolent cancer takes 300 days or more.
- The average size of a breast cancer when first detected by mammography is about 600 million cells, or about 0.25 inches across; the average size detectable by manual palpation is about 45 billion cells and about 1.25 inches in diameter.
- Cancer cells that metastasize exhibit little to no cell-to-cell adhesion as compared to normal cells that tend to adhere to each other to form well-defined tissues (except blood cells).

HOW CANCER BECOMES LIFE-THREATENING

Most cancer deaths are not caused by the direct result of vital organ dysfunction brought on by an encroaching cancerous tumor.

The majority of cancer deaths comes as a result of infection by bacteria, viruses, and fungi – microbes that normally would be destroyed by the immune system. The cancerous body is usually severely immune-compromised because of systemic weakening brought on by the cancer process and partly because of the negative, toxic effects of conventional treatment – chemotherapy, surgery, and radiation.

Severe malnutrition or emaciation may affect up to 90% of all advance cancer patients and account for 50% of all cancer deaths. Cancer cells effectively use up all the body's energy reserves, leaving the body in a dire state of cellular starvation called cachexia. Remember that cancer cells favor glucose as a source of fuel instead of oxygen. Protein-calorie malnutrition is commonly associated with undernourished children in under-developed countries. It is not uncommon among hospitalized patients in general, leading to overall weakness, apathy, increases in mortality and surgical failures, reduced immunity, and poor treatment response.

Signs of Cancer

Cancer can be beaten if you detect it early enough and treat it with natural therapies. These methods work best when the body's tumor is relatively small.

Here are some signs to look for:

- A lump or thickening in the breast or testicles are indicative signs for further investigation.
- A change in a wart or mole may be reflective of melanoma or squamous carcinoma.
- A persistent skin sore that does not heal may be indicative of melanoma.
- A change in bowel or bladder habits, such as constipation, chronic diarrhea, abdominal pain, rectal or urinary bleeding indicating gastrointestinal cancer.
- A persistent cough or coughing up blood, indicating bronchial tree damage.
- Constant indigestion or trouble swallowing, are common signs of colon, stomach, or esophagus cancer.
- Unexplained weight loss, as cancer cells use up your energy source without you knowing it.
- Unusual bleeding or vaginal discharge may be signs of uterine, endometrial or cervical cancer.
- Chronic fatigue, a symptom often accompanied by rapidly progressing cancers.

Cancer is a disease process in which healthy cells stop functioning and maturing properly. Most often triggered and started because of DNA mutation, the end result is the same. There is an accelerated process of inappropriate uncontrolled cell growth – a chaotic process that is abnormal. Cancerous cells represent the summation of the body's response to a continuous attack on its balancing and regulatory mechanisms by over 30 known factors and countless more. According to Jesse Stroff, MD, noted alternative cancer specialist, *"The tumor is not part of the human organism, but represents a rebellion of the cells against the human organism. Consequently, cancer should be considered a disease of the whole organism, not a disease of cells."*

On a simplistic level, cancer can be viewed as the result of a gradual systemic poisoning and weakening of the body's immune system by a multiplicity of stress factors collectively known as carcinogens. These carcinogens, used in a broad sense here for the sake of easy understanding, include chemicals, electromagnetic energy, a faulty diet, free radicals, genetic disposition, toxic metal buildup, radiation, parasites, viruses, and emotional stress, just to name a few. It is the summation of all these carcinogens and immune-suppressing agents acting collectively on our biochemical and psychological makeup that facilitates cancer cell development.

AVOIDING THE RISKS

Most cancer patients are surprised when they are first diagnosed. They know of friends and relatives who have cancer, but normally don't think of themselves as a candidate as well. Why?

After billions of dollars spent on research, we now know that cancer is not a mysterious disease that "just happens" locally with a lump but one with relatively good predictability of occurrence if key contributing factors are identified. Contrary to popular believe, there is a mountain of information on why we get cancer, why certain people are prone to getting it, while others can smoke all their life and not get cancer.

First, you may wish to answer the following questions:

- Do you have fast food more than twice a week?
- Have you been leading a sedentary lifestyle for years?
- Are you happy?
- Do you eat lots of meat and chicken?
- Do you live near a nuclear power plant?

Yes these are all relevant questions, for science has shown their relevance beyond the shadow of doubt. Gone are the days where we think that tobacco smoke MAY lead to cancer as the tobacco companies want us to believe. We now know that first and second hand smoke causes cancer. End of story.

Understanding why cancer happens to some and not others is critical. There are reasons, and if you only look hard, chances are that you will find some, if not all the reasons. You just have to look hard enough.

Many interdependent factors – at least 30 and growing – in various combinations contribute to the development of cancer. Although some cancers have a strong genetic predisposition, and others may be linked to an infectious process; many environmental and psychological factors also come into play.

16 REASONS WHY YOU GET CANCER

Let us look at 16 major proven cancer risk factors that we know of today. The more of these risk factors you are exposed to, the higher your risk. It is never too late to reduce your risk because the toxic effect of carcinogens is cumulative. If you already have been diagnosed with cancer, it is critical that you reduce these factors as quickly as possible to prevent further damage.

1. Sunlight

Solar radiation is responsible for over 400,000 skin cancers a year in the US alone. In particular, ultraviolet-B and C radiations are most damaging. Scientists believe that the ultraviolet component of sunlight induces permanent mutational damage to the DNA of skin cells, affecting a single gene called the p53 tumor suppressor gene. With the depletion of the protective ozone layer more ultraviolet radiation is present than ever before. Three main types of skin cancers are involved: melanoma, squamous cell carcinoma, and basal cell carcinoma.

Risk Reduction Refraining from excessive exposure to direct sunlight. Apply **sunscreens** if you are exposed. But don't forget that 30-45 minutes of exposure to sunshine per week is needed for optimum health.

2. Chronic Exposure to Electromagnetic Fields (EMFs)

Electromagnetic fields are energy fields that in turn have a magnetic effect on their surroundings. They are produced by various sources one of which is electricity. EMFs are part of nature and are radiated by the human body and its organs too. They are also generated by man-made devices such as computer terminals, microwave ovens, overhead lights, electrical poles, and motors, just to name a few. Food mixers, hair dryers, and vacuum cleaners emit EMFs that are 30 to 100 times greater than the suggested safe limit. In fact, ordinary household appliances such as cellular phones, television sets, and electrical outlets tend to generate larger cumulative EMF exposures than power lines because most people are much nearer to these appliances. Although EMFs from appliances drop off at a distance of about 16 feet, people often stand or sit closer than this to the source in the case of household appliances. EMFs interact with living systems, affecting enzymes related to hormonal metabolism, cell division, and gene expression. The frequency of the EMF determines its potency and harmful potential. The frequency of the electric current used in homes in the US is 60 Hz (hertz or cycles per second). In contrast, the ideal frequency of the human brain during waking hours ranges from 8 to 20 Hz, while in sleep, the frequencies may drop to as low as 2 Hz. It is postulated that higher frequencies may disturb the brains' natural resonant frequencies, leading to cellular fatigue and activation of oncogenes. Studies have shown that children living in proximity to large power lines have twice the risk for all cancers, 2.5 times the risk for brain cancer, and three times the risk for leukemia, and the incidence is directly proportional to the amount of time spent exposed to EMF. **Among adults, there is a strong association between EMFs and brain cancer, and, to a less extent,** breast cancer. We do know that melatonin production is reduced in those afflicted with breast cancer, and excessive exposure to weak EMF can disturb the brain's production of melatonin. In fact, a University of North Carolina research team has shown that female electrical workers were 40% more likely to die from breast cancer than women in other occupations.

Risk Reduction **Stay away from EMF as much as possible.** Remove electrical appliances from your bedroom, including electric alarm clocks. Do not use electric blankets, and sleep in a room without a night light. From the workplace or home, get a gauss meter and measure the amount of EMF exposure. Upgrade your electrical circuitry if needed to reduce EMF exposure. Do not use microwave ovens, and stay at least 12 feet away from a TV screen.

3. Ionizing Radiation

Ionizing radiation, such as **X-rays,** consists of high-energy rays that can disrupt the electron from matter, causing genetic mutations that can lead to cancer. Radiologists have historically a higher incidence of cancer, as have other workers exposed to low-dose radiation. X-rays (or gamma rays) also emanate from fluorescent lights, computer monitors, and television screens.

Medical X-rays may be responsible for many breast cancers, according to estimates by John Gofman, MD, PhD, professor emeritus in the department of Molecular and Cell Biology at the University of California at Berkeley. Dr Gofman felt that all kinds of cancer can be induced by radiation, with its effect often felt only decades after the initial exposure. The longer the radiation exposure, the smaller the dose needed to do damage. He announced that the official estimates on cancer risk of radiation exposure had been underestimated by 10 times. These estimates threatened the nuclear power industry, and Dr Gofman was dismissed from his job. The key to preventing cancer, according to Dr Gofman, is elimination of high dose of breast irradiation, including mammogram.

Risk Reduction **Avoid X-rays or mammograms** unless necessary.

4. Pesticide/Herbicide Residues

The widespread use of pesticide is staggering. Ten times as much pesticides are used today compared to 50 years ago. Over 400 pesticides are currently licensed for use on America's food sources. Over 1.2 billion pounds were dumped on crops, land, forests, lawns, and fields. Over 35,000 different formulations of pesticides have come into use over the past five decades worldwide. Some are banned (such as DDT), but many of these eventually find their way to developing countries where they enter the food chain and eventually find their way back to the US as coffee, fruits, and vegetables.

In addition to foods, pesticides are used in building materials (wood preservatives), food containers, golf courses, and parks, just to name a few. Pesticides also leach into the water supply. Many cancer-causing pesticides and industrial chemicals accumulate in fatty tissues of fish, cattle, and poultry. This process of bioaccumulation affects the brain, sexual organs, and breasts because these are organs with the highest concentration of fatty tissue. Unfortunately, less than 1% of all foods are being tested for pesticide residues. There is essentially no escape.

The evidence is clear that **pesticides cause cancer** among farmers and agricultural workers at high doses, including non-Hodgkin's lymphoma. Israel is one of the first countries to ban many toxic chemicals such as DDT and PCBs. In the 10 years since the ban, the rate of breast cancer deaths has declined sharply, with a mortality rate reduction of 30% in women under 44 years old. Pesticides used in the home and garden have been linked to a variety of cancers, including childhood leukemia and brain cancer.

A study done in 1973 by the Hebrew University-Hadassah Medical School in Jerusalem analyzed some tumor samples. The researchers found that when cancerous breast tissue was compared with non-cancerous tissue from elsewhere in the same woman's body, the concentration of toxic chemicals such as DDT and PCBs was "much increased in the malignant tissue compared to the normal breast and adjacent adipose [fat] tissue." Following a public outcry, Israel banned these chemicals from being used on feed for dairy and meat cattle. Over the next 10 years, the rate of breast cancer deaths in Israel declined sharply, with a 30% drop in mortality for women under 44 years of age, and an 8% overall decline. At the same time, all other known cancer risks –alcohol consumption, fat intake, lack of fruits and vegetables in the diet – increased significantly. During this period, worldwide death rates from cancer increased by 4%.

The only answer scientists could find to explain this was the reduced level of carcinogenic environmental toxins.

Risk Reduction   **Eat certified organically grown whole food.**

5. Industrial Toxins

Highly toxic chemicals and heavy metals used in industries often find their way into our body. Such compounds include lead (from **cigarette smoke, ceramic glazes on cooking utensils, canned food), mercury (from dental fillings, fish) aluminium (from antacids, over-the-counter drugs and douches), nickel and cadmium (from cigarettes, instant coffee and teas, nickel-cadmium batteries).** They have a tendency to accumulate in the fat cells, affecting the central nervous system, brain, and glands.

Many environmental chemicals mimic the activity of estrogen once inside the body due to their close resemblance in chemical structure to estrogen; for this reason, they are also called xenoestrogens. They are now believed to contribute to the rising incidence of breast cancer and its epidemic worldwide. Toxins also become synergistically more toxic when combined. For example, combining the normally weak environmental estrogens such as dieldrin and endosulfan results in a compound that is 1,000 times more potent.

The National Academy of Science tells us that the average American ingests 40 mg of pesticides alone and carries about one-tenth of a gram permanently stored in body fat. The average American, regardless of place of residence, is expected to have over 250 chemical contaminants in the body that is verifiable by blood tests.

Risk Reduction   **Avoid smoke** filled environments; avoid fresh and coastal water fish. **Remove any mercury fillings; avoid antacids. Use organic shampoos and toothpastes.**

6. Polluted, Chlorinated and Fluoridated Water

According to the Environmental Protection Agency, the tap water of 30 million Americans contains potentially hazardous levels of lead. One out of every four public water systems has violated Federal standards for tap water. The contaminants include bacteria, radioactive particles, heavy metals, chemical residues, and industrial wastes. Ground water also contains toxic amounts of radionuclides that can cause cancer.

Chlorinated water consumption is linked with a 20-40% increase in the incidence of colon and rectal cancer. In a study conducted by Harvard University and the Medical College of Wisconsin, the consumption of chlorinated drinking water accounts for 15% of all rectal cancers and 9% of all bladder cancers in America. The risk of getting rectal cancer is increased by 38% and bladder cancer by 21% for people drinking chlorinated water.

Fluoridated water, touted as the best way to reduce dental cavity, has been associated with a six times increase in bone cancer in males under age 20. As little as 1 ppm (parts per million) of fluoride in water was found to increase the tumor growth rate in mice by 25%. The incidence of oral and pharyngeal cancer rises with increased exposure to fluoride by as much as 50% accordingly to a study conducted by the National Cancer Institute. The legal limit in the US is 4 ppm. Fluoridated water has been outlawed in most European countries, with no resultant increase in dental decay.

Risk Reduction **Avoid tap water. Drink only pure filtered water.**

7. Tobacco

Over 2,000 chemical compounds are generated by tobacco smoke, many of them poisonous. Over 350,000 deaths occur each year in the US as a result of tobacco use, and 33% of these deaths occur from smoking-related lung cancer alone. In fact, lung cancer can be reduced by 90% if smoking is prohibited. Second hand smoke contains dangerous carcinogens as well, including benzene, radon, and asbestos. It is estimated that 20% of lung cancers are caused by second hand smoke. Smoking increases harmful free radicals and lower our immune system by suppressing the natural killer (NK) cells and IgA (Immunoglobulin A) antibodies. Tar, formed when organic compound is burned, is a leading cancer-causing compound found in tobacco. It contains highly toxic hydrocarbons and some radioactive compounds like potassium-40 as well. These substances have been shown on a cellular basis to damage a tumor suppressor gene called p53 in lung cells, resulting in cancer. Carbon monoxide released during smoking reduces the oxygen supply to the brain, lung and heart. Smokers also have a lower circulating level of vitamin C, an important antioxidant that mops up free radicals.

Risk Reduction **Stay as far away from first and second hand smoke as much as possible.** Take vitamin C for its antioxidant effect against harmful free radicals of tobacco smoke.

8. Hormone Therapies

If you study all the non-genetically linked risk factors associated with breast cancer, it is evident that almost all of them are directly or indirectly associated with an excess of the female hormone estrogen or a relative dominance of estrogen due to progesterone deficiency.

For example, the age at which a woman starts menstruating and the age at which she enters menopause are a proven indicator of risk, and these are dependent on hormone levels. A recent study reported in the Journal of the American Medical Association showed that women who took hormone replacement therapy (HRT) five years or more had an increased breast cancer risk of 1.6 to 1.85 times than women who never took hormones. In the famous Harvard Nurse Study of 1976-1992, it was shown that women in the 55-59 age group who went on estrogen replacement therapy (ERT) for five years or more had a 40% higher risk of developing breast cancer; among women aged 60-64, the risk was 70% higher.

As early as the 1960s, researchers have been sounding the caution bell against the indiscriminate use of estrogen in a hormone replacement therapy program. The average incubation time from cellular damage to full blown cancer is about 20 years. There is very little doubt now that we are in the midst of a breast cancer epidemic worldwide started some 30 years ago, coinciding with the introduction of widespread estrogen use in a hormone replacement program.

Similarly, studies have shown that women who started taking birth control pills under the age of 18 had a three-fold risk of developing breast cancer. Women who took birth control pills for more than four years were twice as likely as non-users to develop breast cancer at age 50.

Risk Reduction Unfortunately, there is no way to escape the estrogen dominant society we are in. In addition to the hormones we take as prescribed by our doctors, environmental estrogens such as plastics or pesticides, enter our body. Sources range from the food we eat to the household cleaning materials we use. There is simply no escape. To reduce your risk, **use organic household supplies; take organic meat free of hormones and free range poultry. Balance estrogen dominance with natural progesterone cream and phytoestrogen-laced vegetables.** Avoid environmental estrogens, such as pesticides, and medicines containing estrogens, such as HRT and Tamoxifen unless absolutely necessary.

9. Wrong Diet and Nutrition

Excessive intake of animal protein has been linked to increased risk of breast, colon, pancreatic, kidney, prostate, and endometrial cancer. Protein is broken down into nitrogenous waste that may be converted into carcinogenic compounds, nitrosamines and ammonium salts. Excessive protein contributes to an acidic terrain and causes a large amount of calcium to leach from bones in an attempt to neutralize such an acidic environment. A chronic acidic environment eventually leads to the loss of calcium resulting in osteoporosis. Large studies have been conducted showing that men who ate red meat over a 5-year period were almost three times more likely to contract advance prostate cancer compared to men who are mainly vegetarians. On a worldwide basis, countries with the fattiest diets also have the highest rate of breast, colon, and prostate cancer. Smoked and pickled meat is also associated with a higher incidence of stomach and esophageal cancer. **Contaminated fresh water fish should be avoided because of potential intoxication. Deep-water fish such as salmon, tuna, red snapper and flounder are generally safe.**

Excessive fat intake, especially animal fat, has been especially associated with higher rates of breast, colon, rectum, uterus, and prostate cancer. Partially hydrogenated vegetable oil (also called trans-fat) commonly found in processed food further contributes to the problem. Most of the fatty acids that we consume from processed food, with the exception of fish, are from the omega-6 class. They are also found in most plant oils such as corn and safflower oils. Excessive omega-6 fats are carcinogenic, while omega-3 fats (found in deep-water and cold-water fish and flaxseed) are beneficial to human health.

An excessive intake of refined carbohydrate and sugar weakens the immune system. Eating only three ounces of sugar in one sitting can reduce the activity of white blood cell by 40%. Sugar is also an ideal environment that cancer cells strive in.

Common foods such as French fries are no better. In a recent study carried out at Stockholm University jointly with Sweden's National Food Administration, a government food safety agency, researchers explained that heating of carbohydrate-rich foods, such as potatoes, rice or cereals formed acrylamide, a human carcinogen. The research was deemed so urgent and important that the scientists decided on the unusual step of releasing it to the press so as to warn the general public before the results were even officially published in an academic journal.

French fries sold at everyone's favorite fast-food restaurants such as Burger King and McDonald contained about 100 times the 1-mcg/liter maximum permitted by the World Health Organization for acrylamides in drinking water. (One mg or 0.001 grams, is equivalent to 1,000 micrograms). Furthermore, an ordinary bag of potato chips contains up to 500 times too much acrylamide using these same criteria set by the WHO. This information certainly sounds very scary.

Fast-food French fries showed the highest levels of acrylamide among the foods tested by an independent agency, Center for Science in the Public Interest (CSPI). CSPI had tested and found that large orders contained 39 to 72 mcg. One-ounce portions of Pringles potato crisps contained about 25 mcg, whereas corn-based Fritos and Tostitos contained half that amount or less. Regular and Honey Nut Cheerios contained 6 or 7 mcg of the carcinogenic substance.

Risk Reduction **Reduce refined sugar and trans-fat intake.** Supplement with optimum doses of nutritional supplements. Focus on plant-based proteins such as beans and legumes, green leafy vegetables, and deep- and cold-water fish for its rich omega-3 content. Think twice before you reach for the potato chips, French fries or other fast foods.

10. Emotional Stress

Under emotional stress, an anti-inflammatory hormone called cortisol is secreted by the adrenal gland commanded by the brain. This hormone weakens the immune system. Chronic stress leads to reduced white blood cell activities and a decreased amount of lymphocytes, causing the thymus gland to shrink. High levels of emotional stress increase one's susceptibility to illness. Studies have shown, for example, that the risk of developing breast cancer was five times higher in women who had experienced an important emotional loss in the six years prior to the discovery of the tumor.

Depression has also been linked to an increased risk of cancer. Loners are 16 times more prone to develop cancer than those who openly discuss their feeling according to a longitudinal study spanning three decades.

Risk Reduction Learn to let go and try meditation to reduce emotional stress. Join a cancer support group and share your worries with others. It is encouraging to know that studies show that cancer survival is increased by an average of 18 months for those who are active participants in a cancer support group.

11. Intestinal Toxicity and Digestive Impairment

An adult's intestines are over 25 feet long when stretched out. Food has to pass through this system during digestion. The undigested food is passed out as excrement. Many believe that optimum health begins with a good digestive tract. A toxic bowel equals a toxic body. Only a century ago, the average transit time from the time food is ingested to the time it is excreted, was 20 hours. Today, some people have transit times of up to 72 hours. The longer food stays in the intestinal tract, the more it putrefies, creating an ideal environment for bacteria to flourish, leading to a myriad of diseases including mal-absorption syndrome, inflammatory diseases, and cancer.

Mucous-producing foods such as milk products and fowl, contribute the most to constipation. On the other hand, fruits and vegetables break down the mucous leading to a faster transit time and less constipation. Mucous, in addition to reducing the absorption power of the intestine, also leads to an imbalance of good and bad flora in the gut. The result is a toxic bowel, with toxins leaching out of the intestine into other tissues. The progressive decrease in hydrochloric acid, pepsin, and pancreatic enzyme also results in poorly digested protein, another source of toxins, not to mention the reduced production of key protein substances such as peptide neurotransmitters for optimum health due to the lack of substrate constituents.

Risk Reduction **Take lots of fiber, green food, and digestive enzyme.** Supplement with fiber and probiotics should be considered.

12. Viruses

It is well known that viruses can cause cancer. Human *papilloma* virus types 16 and 18 have been shown to cause cervical cancer. Hepatitis B virus is also linked to liver cancer. Epstein-Barr virus is linked to about 50% of cancers of the upper pharynx, 30% of Hodgkin's, and 10% of non-Hodgkin's and selected gastric cancers. It is estimated that up to 15% of cancer deaths are due to viruses, bacteria, and parasites.

Risk Reduction **Maintain a strong immune system** with medicinal mushrooms, herbs, exercise, and a low-sugar diet.

13. Blocked Detoxification Pathway

Our immune system does not have an unlimited capacity to fight carcinogens and unwanted bacteria. The body's detoxification system, especially the liver, is a critical component for eliminating toxins and preventing illness. A blocked or sluggish detoxification system increases our susceptibility to cancer. Environment and lifestyle factors can lead to the body being overloaded with metabolic by-products (such as drugs, smoke, chemical additives, and heavy metal), hormonal by-products (such as estrogen-like compounds and growth hormone derivatives from commercial cattle and poultry), free radical by-products (such as tobacco smoke, nuclear and ultraviolet radiation, and excessive exercise), and immune by-products (such as food allergies). Since the liver is a critical organ in the detoxification process, a compromised liver is an invitation to cancer.

Risk Reduction   **Enhance liver function** with herbs such as milk thistle.

14. Cellular Oxygen Deficiency

Cancer cells can live without oxygen, while normal cells cannot. The discovery of this fundamental difference has had a tremendous impact in cancer research. Dr Otto Warburg won his first Nobel Price in 1931 for this discovery. In fact, Dr Warburg was able to show that when you put normal cells from the embryo in an environment devoid of oxygen, they will transform themselves into cancerous cells through the elimination of their prime nutrient. The cell becomes dependent on the fermentation rather than oxidation of glucose for energy. This is an adaptation in order to survive. But the fermentation process is highly inefficient, as a large amount of lactic acid is produced as a by-product. Lactic acid in turn increases the acidity of the body, making it difficult for normal cells to use oxygen.

Cancerous tumors may contain 10 times more lactic acid than healthy human tissues.

Moreover, over the past century, the amount of oxygen we breathe in has diminished. Exposure to tobacco smoke, auto exhaust, and factory emission, the lack of exercise, and shallow breathing all lead to a reduced oxygen supply and an increased carbon monoxide intake. If sufficient oxygen is provided, glucose fermentation stops and normal aerobic respiration returns.

Risk Reduction **Moderate level of aerobic exercise** is absolutely needed to keep the body well oxygenated.

15. Cellular Terrain

If you believe that the body is a closed ecosystem capable of maintaining itself in optimum function, it is logical to deduce that a change in this ecosystem (or internal terrain as some prefer to call it) affects the environment in which organisms grow or die. Factors that modulate the internal terrain include a proper balance of acids and alkalis, and good and bad bacteria, among others. In addition to the Monomorphism Theory advanced by Louis Pasteur, where it is postulated that bacteria maintain one shape and invade the body from the outside causing disease, we now know that certain microbes – a bacterium, fungus, virus, or cell-wall deficient protein material – can change and take on many different shapes that are increasingly pathogenic if the internal terrain is favorable to the microbe. This is called the Polymorphism Theory. In other words, sickness is not so much caused by the microbes, but rather the microbes flourish with the sickness. These deadly agents and cancer only develop if the internal terrain is compromised, such as when it is too acidic. If the internal terrain is balanced, diseases cannot take place.

`Risk Reduction` **Avoid red meat, caffeine containing beverages such as coffee or tea, sugar and dairy foods** which are acidic in nature. Focus on green leafy vegetables that are alkaline in nature. Drink pure filtered water with lemon. Maintain a balanced internal terrain with enzymes, probiotics, fibers, and green food.

16. Genetic Factors

Numerous genes with direct links to cancer have been discovered in recent years. Women with a defect of the BRCA1 tumor suppressor gene, for example, have up to a 80% higher chance of getting breast cancer.

Numerous oncogenes have also been discovered that have the ability to transform normal cells into cancer cells. Numerous external factors including aflatoxins (commonly found in peanuts), electromagnetic radiation (X-rays, sunlight, nuclear radiation), viruses, and hormones, can stimulate such oncogenes.

`Risk Reduction` **Genetic testing** is available and can be considered for early detection. A radical preventive approach is prophylactic mastectomy followed by breast reconstruction surgery for those with proven genetically positive traits.

SUMMARY

Most of us will find it hard to escape from most of the cancer risk factors mentioned. Is there any surprise that the cancer rate worldwide is skyrocketing?

Jesse Stoff, MD, past editor of Journal of Anthroposophic Medicine and author of *Chronic Fatigue Syndrome: The Hidden Epidemic,* sums it up best by saying: *"The tumor is not a part of human organism, but represents a rebellion of the cells against the human organism.*

Cancer should be considered a disease of the whole organism, not a disease of cells." In the past 150 years, we have been misguided to think that cancer is a localized disease of dysfunctional cells. In reality, cancer represents a generalized dysfunctional state with local manifestations.

The key to understanding cancer is to accept the reality that it is a multi-factorial problem and the symptom of a chronic pattern of insults to the body's ecosystem that has gone on for decades. Cancer is not a single cause-and-effect phenomenon at all. It is a collage of symptoms. This foundational understanding will lead us to formulate the kind of natural medicine required to address each of these risk factors and symptoms to bring homeostasis back to the body the way it is supposed to be, and ultimately, to assist the body to reverse cancer naturally.

CHAPTER THREE

NATURAL MEDICINE

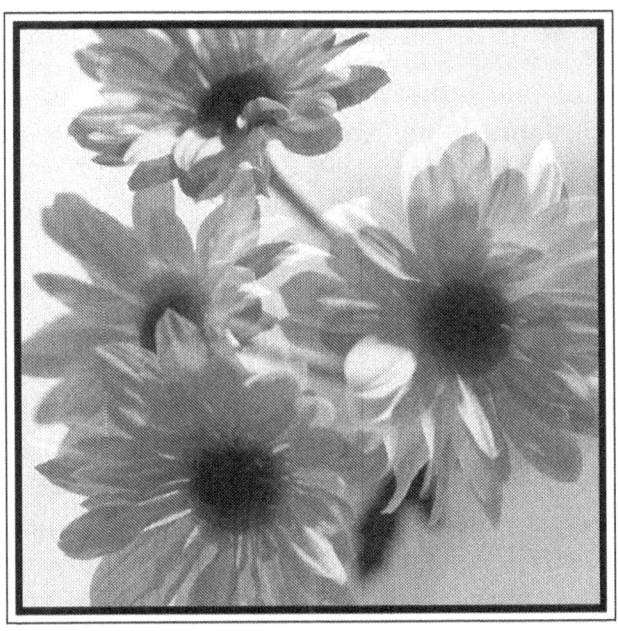

"Just because data are not available does not mean
an alternative treatment is ineffective,
only that we don't yet know."

Dean Ornish, MD, Clinical Professor of Medicine,
University of California, San Francisco, in the book
Breast Cancer – Beyond Convention

C onventional medicine really is NOT traditional at all if you look at the broader perspective from a medical history point of view. This type of medical paradigm worldwide is really a just form of "alternative medicine" that relies on chemicals and surgery to treat illness. Its history is only about 150 years old. It is a wonderful model for acute illness. It is a poor model to follow in treating chronic degenerative diseases, including atherosclerosis and many types of cancer.

What conventional medicine calls "alternative medicine" is actually the true traditional medicine. **Natural therapies are the most common form of medical therapy in the world today, despite the advent of allopathic medicine.** They have been used for thousands of years. They are NOT the alternative but the real medicine suppressed for the past century but now being re-discovered in the West.

Natural medicine is a system of medicine that focuses on prevention and the use of non-toxic natural therapies to restore optimum health.

The natural-oriented physician addresses the patient as one inseparable unit, believing that the body and mind are interconnected. The emphasis is on elimination of underlying causes through the right diet, lifestyle, natural remedies, and preventive measures. The natural physician believes that caring and empathy are critical to healing, that the physician is a partner in the healing process; and that the patient is in charge of health-care choices.

The biggest difference is that allopathic medicine tends to view good health as a physical state in which there is no obvious disease present, while the natural physician recognizes true health as an optimal state of physical, mental, emotional, and spiritual well-being.

How does this relate to cancer? Let us zoom in.

CANCER ACCORDING TO NATURAL MEDICINE

The person gets cancer because he's not properly metabolizing the protein in his diet.
— Dr Kelley, of the famed Kelley Anti-cancer Therapy

Modern oncology (the study of tumors) is founded on the Halstead Theory of Cancer developed by W.S. Halstead who lived from 1852-1922. The central premise here about cancer is that the tumor is virtually considered the living organism and not the patient. Under this hypothesis, the removal of a tumor should remove the disease and cure the patient. If this theory were true, why is it that the age-adjusted mortality rate for breast cancer has remained virtually unchanged for the past 50 years despite advances in surgical techniques and aggressive cancer debulking operations? Halstead's theory is flawed because it emphasizes the tumor and ignores the patient. He looked at the tumor as the disease in and of itself, disregarding the overall body as the contributing factor. This hypothesis is clearly wrong.

While conventional medicine primarily treats cancer as a focal disease with localized symptoms, natural-oriented physicians think otherwise. Natural-oriented physicians think of the body as a closed internal ecosystem, and believes that it is the dysfunction of this ecosystem that is primarily responsible for the development of cancer.

No treatment, conventional or otherwise, can completely eliminate all cancer cells according to natural medicine. The reason is simple. Cancer is a systemic disease, and there are simply too many cancerous or pro-cancerous cells within the ecosystem of the body. Cancer is not a localized problem but a whole-body phenomenon of metastatic growth. Its growth process is affected by biological conditions. Non-genetically-based cancer forms in the body because of toxins, the lack of oxygen, poor nutrition, and other factors such as hormonal imbalance. Whether the cancer in our body continues to multiply depends to a large degree on our body's biological terrain. It is this terrain that determines how the cancer is expressed.

Natural-oriented doctors view cancer as a chronic, systemic and metabolic dysfunction of the intracellular genetic makeup. Tumors are only the symptoms of the sub-microscopic dysfunctional causes.

The natural medicine therefore fights cancer by optimizing the internal terrain and enabling the patient's internal system to destroy the tumor. It enhances the patient's health so that cancer cells cannot grow and multiply.

Now let us look at an example of how breast cancer is treated differently by conventional and natural medicine. Conventional doctors focus on the breast tissue itself. He will recommend the patient to undergo surgery, chemotherapy, or radiological therapy directed at the breast mass. A natural-oriented physician will look at breast cancer as a symptom of underlying hormonal imbalance and will attempt to rid the cancer by rebalancing the hormonal system. The most ideal treatment for the patient will be to integrate both conventional and natural medicine to remove the growth and underlying imbalance of hormones.

Basis of Natural Medicine

Non-toxic therapies used in natural medicine have been proven to prevent cancer metastases. They can be used as an adjunct to and sometimes even as a better replacement for conventional therapies because they are not toxic and do not have any significant undesirable side effects. Now, let us take a closer look at the science behind some of these natural therapies.

As we have seen earlier, cancer cells have characteristics that are different from normal cells. They thrive in high-sugar and acidic environments and are killed at a temperature of 43°C. They are inefficient generators of energy. Instead of using oxygen to oxidize glucose as the primary fuel source and putting out carbon dioxide as normal cells do, they prefer to ferment sugar as a source of energy and produce lactic acid as waste. Non-toxic natural therapies focus on overcoming cancer by helping the body create an internal environment that is unfavorable to cancer cell function.

There are thousands of natural therapies used to treat cancer. How do you know which one is good? Modern day science dictates that any treatment, natural or conventional, must conform to the following criteria before one should embark on it. Otherwise, it is better classified as "quackery".

1. There must be science to justify its use objectively.
2. Some form of mechanism of action must be known.
3. The therapy cannot be toxic to the body.
4. The therapy should not interfere with chemotherapy or radiotherapy.
5. They must be suitable for long-term therapy.
6. They are active at concentrations that are achievable in humans.

No amount of evidence can convince the skeptical mind. Science is an art that progresses through time. When the tomato was first discovered, the scientific community unanimously agreed that the red color was indeed a sign of toxicity. For 500 years, the tomato was labeled a toxic food and not eaten. That was science. Similarly, the doctor who advocated that surgeons should wash their hands before going into surgery, was expelled from the hospital for introducing the "unscientific" idea at that time. That was also science.

Let us look at some more interesting "science". Some 40 years ago, Dr Linus Pauling, a two time Nobel laureate postulated that taking vitamin C as a supplement could extend one's life. He was so excited that he put forth this idea to the public. Too bad, nobody believed him. The mainstream medical community ridiculed his "cock-and-bull" story. Nevertheless, he continued faithfully to take vitamin C on a daily basis. He passed away at the ripe age of 94 and contributed the last 18 years of his life to this supplement intake. Now, 40 years later, it is a widely accepted fact that free radicals cause mutational damage and is a primary cause of cancer. Vitamin C counteracts such free radicals. It took a good 30 years before the medical community started paying attention to his theory. Many more lives could have been saved if only the people had put their trust in him earlier.

When does science becomes accepted? Unfortunately, science becomes science when the majority of scientists accepts it.

"Discovery is seeing what everyone saw and thinking about what no one thought", Albert Szent-Gyoergy, Nobel laureate and discoverer of vitamin C, said. The essence of the statement is that few in the world would know, understand, or accept what is new. New truths go through three stages. First they are ridiculed, then they are violently opposed, and finally, they are accepted as being "self-evident". How long does it take? Anywhere from 40 to 500 years, as we have seen earlier. In the case of cancer, when we are dealing with survival times in days and months, and few cancer patients can afford to wait more than a few weeks.

Not all natural therapies are useful for cancer. They may be good for other ailments but ineffective for cancer. While embracing scientifically proven natural therapies, we must proceed with care to weed out those natural therapies that are less sound or ineffective. Good scientists and clinicians alike focus on those therapies with the most scientific data, knowing full well that in certain cases we only have a "best guess scenario" at this infant stage of our knowledge. Indeed, solid long-term double-blind data required by modern science to validate some natural therapies are still decades away. We are in a race against time in the case of cancer, and often times for humanitarian reasons, we simply do not have the time to wait. The key is to at least "do no harm" to the patient. That much, we have a burden to uphold.

At the end, the burden of proceeding with natural medicine as an adjunct to or in place of conventional therapy rests with the patient and his or her oncologist. Blessed are those who have access to someone knowledgeable in both areas and are able to make an informed decision based on the latest available data.

Uses of Natural Medicine

The main objectives of using natural therapies are:

1. Primary prevention of cancer. This is important for those who have a strong family history of cancer.
2. Secondary prevention. More than eight million patients in the United States alone have been diagnosed with cancer where the cancer is now in remission. Prevention of a recurrence of cancer is therefore the objective for this group of people.
3. To reduce the side effects resulting from conventional therapies such as chemotherapy or radiation therapy.
4. To enhance the body's immunity system.
5. In advanced stages of cancer, when conventional therapies have failed, many patients have no choice but resort to alternative treatments.

You don't need to have diagnosed cancer to be on a natural medicine program. You can do it for prevention of cancer. In fact, those who are proactive or have a family history of cancer would be wise to start an anti-aging and cancer prevention program using natural medicine on a prophylactic basis well ahead of any symptoms of cancer.

How Natural Therapies Fight Cancer

The cancer inhibitory effect of most natural compounds does not directly cause DNA damage, as compared to drugs. Similarly, natural compounds are less likely to cause DNA mutation in surviving cells. In fact, they act selectively on cancer cells without affecting normal cells most of the time.

Specifically, natural compounds fight cancer by:

1. Strengthening the immune system.
2. Preventing the spread of cancer cells through inhibition of angiogenesis or growth of new blood vessels feeding the cancer cells.
3. Creating an environment that is unfavorable for cancer growth. The ideal environment creates a high oxygen level, high metabolism, a high temperature, a low sugar level, and a high alkalinity environment in the body.
4. Detoxifying the body and preventing further toxic buildup in the body.
5. Supporting all targeted organs, especially those affected directly by the cancer.
6. Fighting free radicals that cause mutational changes that lead to cancer formation.

The Natural Medicine Arsenal

There are literally hundreds of non-toxic natural therapies available. Some are well tested while others are purely experimental. The more common ones include:

1. Indictables such as Ukrain, 714X, Mistletoe, Amygladin/Laetrile, oxygenation therapies and tissue extracts.
2. Oral supplementation programs such as vitamins, minerals, enzymes, amino acids, proteins, antioxidants, hormones, pro-hormones, medicinal mushrooms, traditional herbs, glandular extracts and botanicals.
3. Modalities that alter the biological terrain such as hyperthermia, frequency modulation, hyperbaric oxygen, ozone therapy, bio-magnetics, ultraviolet (UV) blood irradiation, insulin induced chemotherapy and detoxification.
4. Psychological support such as counseling, meditation, visualization training and qigong.
5. Dietary and lifestyle adjustments such as Gerson Therapy, macrobiotic or modified macrobiotic diets, vegetarianism, stress reduction and exercise.

NATURAL MEDICINE COCKTAILS

It is true. Cancer patients generally have to take a handful of nutritional supplements. It is not uncommon at all, but is it necessary? Generally speaking, moderate amounts of nutritional supplements are needed to deliver the optimum blend of nutrients to the body. The precise blend and quantity is highly dependent on the natural physician's experience and the patient's condition. Putting together this blend of nutrients in a cancer setting is a highly specialized field of study in itself. It is important to understand that natural medicine works quite differently from drugs. Let us now look at it in more detail.

First, we must understand that cancer-prone events occur in our bodies in clusters. These include:

- Genetic instability in the nucleus
- Abnormal expression of genes, resulting in too few proteins that inhibit cancer and too many that facilitate it
- Abnormal cell-to-cell communications
- Induction of angiogenesis
- Invasion and metastasis
- Immune evasion

Non-toxic natural compounds target these clusters of events and not any one single event. This is a task that no single compound can perform. Fortunately, most natural non-toxic compounds can inhibit several pro-cancer events at the same time. A large combination of natural compounds will target these clusters and at the same time provide a backup for other compounds.

Combining natural compounds into cocktails or blends allow for synergistic interaction. When using natural compounds alone as a single agent, a larger dosage may be required. However, this may lead to higher chances of adverse effects. Therefore, blending the many natural compounds into a manageable cocktail may eliminate these direct-acting side effects and make natural compounds more effective at a lower and safer dosage. For this reason, a nutritional cocktail is often required.

How to Design the Cocktail

Due to the large number of natural compounds available, it is imperative that **a planned approach be adopted** so that the patient is not overwhelmed by the sheer number of compounds that come in the form of powders, tablets, capsules, liquids, or even suppositories.

Here are some parameters on how natural compounds are blended together in a cocktail:

- Using a large number of natural compounds with different target actions to assure redundancy and facilitate synergism. Between 15-30 compounds may be used at a time. For example, use 10 different antioxidants instead of a single one.
- Choose natural compounds that have multiple modes of action. For example, melatonin is an antioxidant as well as hormonal balancer.
- To ensure diversity, choose a few within a large group of similar compounds that have the same desired effect instead of relying on one or two. For example, coenzyme Q10 (or CoQ10) and magnesium both increase the efficacy of the mitochondria. Use both instead of just one or the other.
- Eliminate compounds that are not practical due to dosage or delivery system issues, among others. Powdered shark cartilage, for example, needs to be taken in very high dose for it to work and may not be suitable for many.

The planning of an optimum blend of non-toxic natural compounds and conventional therapies is not simple, as it requires in-depth knowledge of these therapies and extensive clinical experience. Do not try to self-administer as the wrong cocktail could do more harm than good.

What is the Success Rate?

The use of non-toxic natural therapies has achieved huge success over the past few decades. Extensive studies have proven them to have an edge over conventional therapies. Some of the examples are listed below.

Many of the alternative cancer hospitals are found in Mexico. For example, Dr Contreras of the Oasis Hospital reported that his 5-year survival rate for prostate cancer is 83% when using natural treatment compared to 73% for conventional treatment.

In advance-stage bronchogenic carcinoma, natural therapies resulted in an improvement in the quality of life for the patients. Stage IV cancer patients said that their quality of life was better after using the antioxidants. The size of their tumors was reduced by half in some of the cases. Even if their tumor did not subside, the patients felt much better physically.

At the American Metabolic Institute, renowned scientist Dr Geronimo Rubio reported success rates in reversing stage III and IV cancers from 65 to 75%. The reversal rate for stage I and II cancers is 80%.

The famous Gerson Therapy boasted high achievements. In a study spearheaded by Gerson, 153 patients in various stages of melanoma were examined. He was proud to report that all 153 patients who underwent the Gerson Therapy survived for five years. Only 79% of patients who received conventional treatment survived this length of time. Patients with stage IIIA melanoma who underwent Gerson Therapy had a 5-year survival rate of 82% versus 39% in conventional therapy. For stage IIIB, the survival rate was 70% versus 41% in conventional therapy. In stage IVA, the rate was 39% as compared to 6%. These results are simply stunning.

While the 5-year survival for end-stage cancer using conventional therapy is 9% overall, alternative cancer hospitals report that theirs is more than 30%. While 4% of terminal cancer patients show no response to alternative treatments, the other 96% can expect some benefits after a month of treatment. There is therefore no turning back for patients who have bravely embarked on the path of alternative treatments.

In another study published in *Anticancer Research* by Finnish researcher Jaakkola, high doses of nutritional compounds were prescribed along with chemo- and radiation therapies for terminally ill small-cell lung cancer patients. While the 30-month survival rate for advance lung cancer is less than 1%, Jaakkola found that 8 of 18 (44%) were still alive 6 years after therapy.

Dr Hoffer conducted and reported in his book, *Vitamin C and Cancer*, a study of 129 end-stage cancer patients who received concomitant oncology care. The control group of 31 patients who did not receive nutrition support lived an average of less than 6 months. The treated group of 98 cancer patients was divided into 3 groups:

1. 19 were poor-responders. These represent 20% of the treated group. These patients survived an average of 10 months, a 75% improvement over the control group.
2. 47 were good responders. They lived an average of 6 years, a 1,200% improvement over the control group.
3. 32 were good female responders. This group had hormonal imbalance cancers such as cervix, breast, ovary, and uterus. Their average lifespan was over 10 years, or a 2,100% improvement. In fact, many of them were still alive at the end of the study.

In another study, this time by oncologists at West Virginia Medical School, 65 patients with transitional cell carcinoma of the bladder were given either a "one-a-day" vitamin supplement in accordance with the RDA, or a mega-vitamin program consisting the same basic vitamin plus 40,000 IU of vitamin A, 100 mg of vitamin B6, 2,000 mg of vitamin C, 400 IU of vitamin E, and 90 mg of zinc. After 10 months, 80% of the control group (receiving just one-a-day vitamin) had recurrence, while in the mega-dose group, the recurrence of tumor was much lower at 40%. Five-year projected tumor recurrence was 91% for the control group and 41% for the mega-vitamin group.

In other words, high-dose mega-vitamins cut the recurrence rate by almost 50%.

In fact, a study of 200 cancer patients who experienced spontaneous regression showed that 87% of them made major changes in diet, most vegetarian in nature, 55% of them used some form of detoxification, and 65% used nutritional supplements. These are all modalities of natural medicine.

Researchers at Tulane University compared the survival rate of pancreatic cancer patients who either continued with the Western diet or switched to a macrobiotic whole-food diet. Pancreatic cancer is one of the most deadly we know. Of the 1,467 patients tracked, only 10% were alive after one year, while 52% of those who changed their diets were still alive after one year.

Clearly, the success rate of natural treatment, when combined with conventional therapy, is far above that of conventional cancer treatment alone. Today, many patients opt for combination therapy, using both conventional and alternative cancer treatments. This combined therapy is becoming more and more popular as the success rates are high.

Patients in the advance stages of cancer may begin the natural therapy program as soon as the cancer is detected, if time permits. If the natural therapy is not effective, then conventional intervention should be considered. In life-threatening cases where surgical debulking is required, conventional treatment should be used first, followed by natural therapy as part of the healing process.

THREE CANCER STRATEGIES

1. Treat cancer using conventional therapy alone

Conventional therapy works at destroying as many cancer cells as possible. The methods used are surgery, chemotherapy and radiation. Sometimes, a combination of these therapies is used. The objective is to remove the tumor, after which the patient is considered cured.

2. Treat cancer using natural therapy alone

This therapy detoxifies the body and enhances the immunity system so as to immobilize cancer cells. It reverses the process of metastasis through stimulating the body's healing response against the cancer, rather than removing the cancer. The focus is on the whole body and not on the specific cancerous tissues. Very few doctors recommend this and fewer patients opt for this method as the only source of treatment. Yet, some patients have been miraculously cured by this method alone.

This therapy is the most effective for early-stage cancers that have not begun to spread. It also works well in new cases of cancer, where patients have not undergone any forms of conventional treatment yet. Unfortunately, most patients only seek alternative treatment when conventional treatments have failed. By then, many patients are only left with a few months to live. During this critical period, the natural-oriented physician will have not only to work hard at destroying the cancer by boosting their patients' immunity, they also have to fight to overcome the toxic effects of surgery, chemotherapy, and radiation. It is a tough job to handle given the very narrow time frame.

Like in conventional medicine, certain cancers respond better to natural treatments than others. **Cancer of the breast, colon and lungs respond best to natural therapy.** The leukemia and lymphoma families of cancer do moderately well. Cancer with extensive liver metastasis or pancreatic cancer is very difficult to treat both with either conventional or alternative therapy.

3. Combining conventional and natural therapies

This method seeks to destroy as many cancer cells as possible through conventional methods with natural therapies as an adjunct, or vice versa.

The patient is given natural therapies and compounds before, during and after going for the conventional treatments. Detoxification is integrated into part of the overall treatment protocol. The body's immunity is strengthened to prepare it for the negative side effects resulting from the conventional treatments. After conventional treatment, the body will continue to undergo other non-toxic natural therapies to prevent cancer cell recurrence.

Most people choose this option as the most sensible and logical approach.

A. Combining natural therapy and chemotherapy

Human and animal studies have shown successful and amazing results with combined chemotherapeutic agents and natural compounds.

The objectives and rationale behind combining conventional therapies with natural treatments are as follows:

a. To reduce the negative side effects of chemotherapy and radiotherapy so that a more effective and safer dose can be given.

High success rates have been reported in this aspect. Antioxidants such as vitamin C, melatonin and vitamin E have protected animals from drug-induced toxicity without interfering with the drug's anti-tumor effect. It not only protects normal tissues from free radicals caused by chemotherapy but also acts as an immunity booster and produces healthier cells that need a high concentration of antioxidants to function in optimum form.

b. To enhance normal cell resistance to chemotherapy and radiotherapy or increase drug accumulation in cancer cells.

Cancer cells adapt to stress more readily than normal cells. They are much stronger after being exposed to chemotherapy. Natural compounds will destroy the heat-shock proteins that protect the cancer cell. As a result, drug resistance of the cancer cells will be lowered.

c. Additive or synergistic cytotoxic effect with chemotherapy and radiotherapy.

When natural compounds are combined with chemotherapeutic drugs, the cytotoxic effect is additive. Natural compounds and chemotherapy drugs may destroy the cancer cell through different but complementary pathways. The following are examples.

Selenium, a natural supplement, has been proven to reduce both the adverse effects of cisplatin and multi-drug resistance induced by cisplatin. Two grams of vitamin C can enhance the effect of doxorubicin, cisplatin, and paclitaxel against breast cancer cells. In another study, mushroom polysaccharides PSK or PSP have prolonged the lives of tumor-bearing rodents and protected them from the adverse effects caused by chemotherapy.

The natural compound glutamine reduces adverse effects caused by chemotherapy in gastrointestinal-related disease.

Proteolytic enzymes help in absorption and tissue diffusion of drugs, including antibiotics and chemotherapy drugs.

Quercetin and genistein act synergistically with many chemotherapy drugs, including cisplatin. In addition, Green tea, emodin and ginseng also have synergistic effects. However, the dosage administered is often quite high.

Vitamin E enhances the effectiveness of chemotherapy against cancer cells and protects the normal cell.

In a study conducted, vitamin A in the form of retinyl palmitate was used with vitamin C, vitamin E and other minerals in patients with small-cell lung cancer. The consumption of these vitamins actually prolonged the lives of these patients. Their two-year survival rate was increased to 33%, compared with 15% otherwise.

Another natural agent, melatonin, also acts as an antioxidant and reduces the adverse effect of chemotherapy without lessening its anti-tumor actions.

B. Combining natural and radiation therapies

Not much has been researched into this area. More studies are needed to confirm the results on the effectiveness of antioxidants in patients undergoing radiotherapy. However, we are sure of the fact that antioxidants protect patients from some ugly side effects of radiation exposure including ulceration and fibrosis. These effects are often due to inflammatory processes that antioxidants can inhibit. Vitamin E, fish oil and silymarin are particularly helpful in this respect.

DESIGN OF A SUCCESSFUL INTEGRATED PROGRAM

A successful integrated strategy of treating cancer utilizing conventional and non-toxic natural therapies depends on three factors:

1. Data collection

A set of detailed data on each individual cancer patient will have to be compiled. After a thorough study, doctors should use the least toxic therapy first. Strong treatments should only be used as a last resort when other treatments have failed.

The doctor will need to monitor the patient closely. He will use every possible medical and laboratory advancement including PET scans, cancer markers, and immunological studies to detect the presence of cancer and monitor the effectiveness of non-toxic modalities.

2. Selecting the right therapy

The doctor must chart out a comprehensive plan and strategy for the cancer patient based on the data collected. Conventional therapies may be incorporated into the overall plan at strategic points together with non-toxic natural therapies.

There is a large variety of programs that can be offered to the cancer patient. Some of these include antioxidant therapy, dietary changes, modulation of the internal biological terrain, regulation of intestinal balance with probiotics, detoxification of heavy metals with chelation agents, nutritional therapy with supplementation, modulation to enhance the immune function, hormone therapy, antiviral and antimycotic therapies, psychotherapy and physical therapy.

3. Selecting the right timing

In general, patients with advance-stage cancers benefit more from natural therapies than from chemotherapies. As such, cancer patients who are in their advance stages should not be too anxious and should consider postponing chemotherapy if possible. They should try natural therapies first. If this does not work, then perhaps they can go on to try chemotherapy.

Cancer is a process that does not come on overnight. Do not rush into surgery unless there is a life-threatening condition. One should try using the natural approach first as it will only take 4 to 12 weeks to see its effectiveness. It is not that long a time to wait and may be worth it in the long run.

By using natural strategies first, the body's immunity system is strengthened. In early-stage cancers, this approach may be all that is needed to reverse the cancer. It will also prepare the body for the toxic conventional treatments if found to be necessary later.

FOUR PILLARS OF A SUCCESSFUL INTEGRATED ANTI-CANCER PROGRAM

In cancer treatment, there is no magic formula. All programs must be individually tailored to suit the cancer patient as everyone has a different reaction to cancer.

We will now examine the four main components of a successfully integrated cancer strategy.

1. Emotional and Psychological

The state of the mind is an important factor when treating cancer. Patients must think positively. They must have a strong will to live if they want to beat cancer. Meditation and stress reduction counseling from the patient's psychologist, psychiatrist and religion may be helpful. We shall not deal with this in this book.

2. Structural

Natural components address the structural organ function that is the primary site of the disease symptoms. Conventional treatments focus on the cancer growth to rid the body of such structural damage. This component is best dealt with by conventional Western-trained allopathic doctors.

3. Energy

This is the electromagnetic and vibrational energy that flows within the body through various energy pathways called meridians. Disturbance of such meridians is believed to cause organs to dysfunction and lower our body's immunity. This disharmony can be harmonized by using Chinese and Japanese herbs, acupuncture, acupressure, qigong, resonance, magnetic therapy, vibrational therapy and homeopathy. We are still in the infancy stage as far as understanding the potential and power of these modalities is concerned. Empirical clinical data point to their efficacy, although long-term studies are still years away from being conducted. Nevertheless we shall examine some of the most popular ones on the market in later chapters of this book.

4. Biochemical

Chemical analyses of metabolic and energy pathways, hormonal, heavy metal, biological terrain, and mineral status are now readily available to help the cancer patient. We now have about 50 years of scientific data in this area, and the knowledge is growing exponentially. A comprehensive program of nutritional supplementation, diet and detoxification can be tailored for the patient. A doctor who has both Western and Eastern medical backgrounds will be in the best position to deal with this component.

A successful cancer treatment must incorporate the above four components. In the following chapters, we will look into the intricate balancing of the biochemical pathway in a cancer setting. The latter comprises a myriad of related natural therapies. Each focuses on a minute but vital aspect of the overall biochemical function.

IS NATURAL MEDICINE FOR ME?

There are basically two types of patients. One type want their doctor to make the best decision concerning their cancer treatment on their behalf. These patients are not interested in doing their own research. They have faith in the current medical system, and are happy about it. If you fall into this category, then this book is not for you.

The second group of patients like to make their own informed decision based on data supplied by their doctor. They may not be very knowledgeable, but they are willing to learn, to find out, and to make the final decision on treatment options most suited to them. Experience shows that patients with the most success in beating cancer are those that are most involved. Working with their doctor, they learn, ask questions, and take control and responsibility for their body.

But before you even embark on the process of natural healing, it is critical that you ask yourself whether you belong to the first or the second group of patients outlined above.

Let me help you by outlining the three steps you should take to make this critical decision. No one should embark on a natural medicine program without understanding what it is all about. It is easy for those who embark on this journey to fail. It is not easy by any means, the rewards are obvious.

Step 1: Face the reality

Do not deny that you have cancer. All adults do. You just have it more than others. You are not alone, and millions before you have the same. What you have can be beaten. It is not the end of the world. Do not be afraid. Death is a natural consequence of living. Some have to go earlier, while others later. Know that it's the quality of life that counts. Take a moment to focus on the real important issues of life:

- Relationships you cherish
- Your mission in life
- Nature and its beauty
- Being at peace with your Creator

Clear your mind of negative thoughts. Cherish the life you have had and give thanks. The fact that you can even pick up this book to read is a cause for thanksgiving. Many are less fortunate than you. That is a fact.

Do you want to beat cancer? It is done all the time. Those who have the strongest will to live also have the best odds of beating cancer. Tell yourself "I refuse to die!" and list out the reasons why.

Maybe it's your wish to be with your love ones, or you have a mission still not completed. Whatever the reasons may be, list them out. Without a reason to fight, no war can be won. Until your reasons for fighting the war on cancer are clear, do not proceed. Take your time to think it through. Talk to your love ones.

The road to beating cancer requires a change of lifestyle and thinking for many of us. Are you prepared to do what is right instead of what is convenient? Are you prepared to admit the wrongs you have done to your body in the past and take steps to correct them?

Are you prepared to go against the advice of many of your friends or even some doctors? Are you prepared to be labeled as someone who uses "quackery?" Do you seek acceptance, or do you seek well-being?

What is the reward? Is being cancer free a good enough goal for you? If you are a pacifist, it is best to put down the book now and enjoy your remaining days in peace and quiet solitude.

Do not be afraid to say: *"I do not wish to change. I am what I am, and I will accept the consequences."* Blessed are those who know who they are, for that is the true path to happiness. Do not let others tell you why you should or should not fight cancer. The decision is a personal one. There is no right and no wrong to it, and no apology is necessary.

If you have decided that you want to beat cancer, make a commitment, ask for a support group (perhaps your family or close friends), announce your intention, and you are now ready to move on. Incidentally, research has shown that cancer patients who participate actively in a support group live on the average 18 months longer.

You may take days to make this commitment. Do not move to step 2 until you are clear on this step.

Step 2: Do your homework

Fighting a war requires a battle plan together with a general you can trust. Before you can have a plan and appoint your general, you must first understand your battle in its every detail, the desired end result, and the price you are prepared to pay.

Talk to your doctor; get the official medical diagnosis, the staging, and any variance. Search the Internet for as much information as possible on the cancer you can, from both conventional and alternative approaches. Verify that the prognosis and treatment plan advanced by your oncologist conforms to established protocol. Write down on paper, questions you may have on your cancer. The more questions the better.

You need a general and a team in charge to fight this war. Who should they be? Are you comfortable with your current doctor? Do you need a second opinion? Do you need other supporting healthcare professionals such as a nutritionist, and psychotherapist to help you?

This is the time to gather as much knowledge, options, and data as possible. It may entail many phone calls, visits to professionals you have never heard of in distant lands, exploring options that sound like foreign language to you. Yes this is uncharted territory for you, and you need to do your homework as quickly as possible. The good news is that there are professionals out there who can help you, and this is the time to call them.

Do not forget that your commitment from step 1 still stands. You are on track, and you are serious about beating cancer.

Step 3: Make the decision

Chances are your doctor may not be familiar with natural medicine and its role in fighting cancer. Give him a copy of this book and educate him.

Do the concepts advanced by this book make sense scientifically? Go to the library or the Internet. Search for studies on nutritional medicine and verify its effectiveness. Leave no stones unturned. You only have one body, and you cannot afford not to give it the best.

Natural medicine is about lifestyle changes. It is about taking non-toxic food-based supplements in quantity. It is about a new outlook in medicine from the way you have traditionally thought of it. It is about doing things quite differently than what you have been used to. It is 80% mental and 20% physical. Are you ready?

If you have decided to pursue natural medicine as the solution to your cancer, either as an adjunct to or in place of conventional therapy, read on.

CHAPTER FOUR

PREVENT MUTATIONS

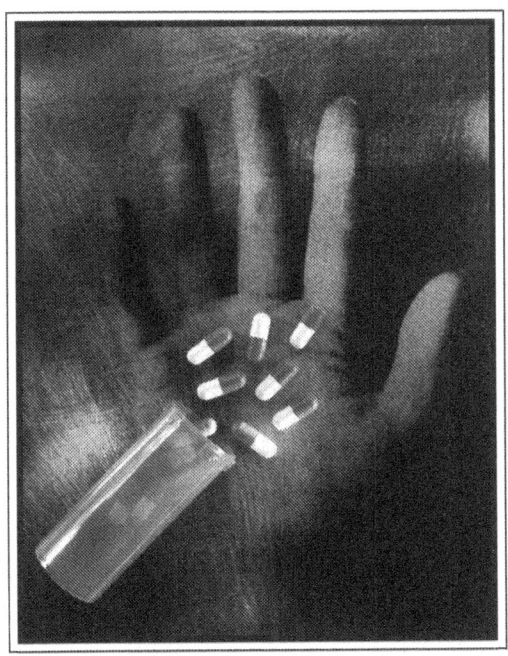

"The integrity of every cell in the body depends on the balance of free radicals and antioxidants."

Stephen Sinatra, MD, cardiologist in his book
Optimum Health

Genes are units of the chromosomes that control our heredity and the destiny of each and every cell in our body. They form the very core of human health.

Changes in genes, more commonly known as genetic mutations, commonly lead to cancer. Such a mutation may be linked to the faulty genes we inherited. More commonly, they are caused by improper dietary habits, unhealthy lifestyles, or environmental pollution brought on ourselves during our own lifetime.

The main agent responsible for mutational changes is called a free radical. Fortunately, free radicals can be neutralized by natural compounds called antioxidants. Research cites that up to 60% of cancer patients are taking antioxidants, with or without the knowledge of their oncologist.

The use of antioxidants as a supplement to conventional therapies plays an important role in natural non-toxic cancer therapy that every natural-oriented cancer patient must be thoroughly familiar with.

FREE RADICALS AND ANTIOXIDANTS

Molecules contain atoms and atoms in turn are made up of a nucleus surrounded by an orbit of electrons. In a stable molecule, these electrons orbit around their respective nuclei in pairs of electrical charges. This gives the molecule a net neutral charge in its stable state. When the molecule is disturbed, it can either lose an electron or gain an extra electron. This results in a molecule with an unpaired electron. Such a charged molecule is called a free radical.

Free radicals are highly reactive. They will try to combine with other molecules in order to steal an electron to return to its stable state. When another molecule loses its electrons to this free radical, it becomes a free radical itself. The process is continuous and self-perpetuating.

Our body's normal metabolic processes produce free radicals. These free radicals are formed as a by-product in the production of ATP (our body's energy currency) from glucose. Some white blood cells destroy invading microbes and in the process produce free radicals. Free radicals are also produced by pollution, cigarette smoke and sunlight.

Too much free radicals in our bodies cause cellular damage. Serious disease such as arthritis, heart disease, cataracts, cancer, Alzheimer's and Parkinson's diseases are linked to a state of excessive free radical activity. Our body's fats, protein,carbohydrates, and DNA can be damaged by free radicals. Tissues and membranes that are exposed to free radical damage lose their ability to properly transport nutrients. Lipoproteins are changed into a dangerous form, resulting in atherosclerosis and damaged DNA causes intracellular mutational changes that lead to cancer.

Antioxidants comprise molecules manufactured by our bodies to remove the effects of free-radical damage. Antioxidants donate an extra electron to the free radical without becoming destabilized itself. As such, it prevents the otherwise self-perpetuating free-radical process.

CLASSES OF ANTIOXIDANTS

There are many types of antioxidants. They can be classified broadly into the following groups:

Antioxidant Enzymes

1. Super Oxide Dismutase
This enzyme contains a highly reactive form of oxygen. It converts the very reactive free radical super oxide into hydrogen peroxide, with zinc and manganese acting as co-factors.

2. Catalase

Hydrogen peroxide is less reactive than super oxide but is still somewhat unstable and able to cause the formation of free radicals. Catalase converts the hydrogen peroxide formed by super oxide dismutase, as well as other super oxides to oxygen and water.

3. Glutathione Peroxidase

Glutathione removes peroxides that contribute to the formation of free radicals. Glutathione peroxidase then converts highly reactive molecules like lipid peroxides into less reactive molecules.

Molecular Antioxidants

4. Vitamin C

Vitamin C, a water-soluble antioxidant that moves around freely within the plasma, helps to recycle vitamin E and other antioxidants. Smoking lowers vitamin C metabolism and plasma thus resulting in high levels of oxidative stress. Vitamin C is essential for building strong immunity and eye health and prevents cancer and heart diseases.

5. Vitamin E

This is a fat-soluble antioxidant that helps prevent oxidation of fatty acids and proteins. The oxidative process can change unprotected LDL-cholesterols. When oxidized, the LDL-cholesterol particles are absorbed by macrophages that lead to the formation of fatty streaks and atherosclerotic plaques. Vitamin E protects LDL particles from oxidation and protects our vascular walls.

6. Carotenoids

These are derived from more than 500 different pigments from plants. Examples are beta-carotene, lutein, lycopene and zeaxanthin. Carotenoids function in a different way. They act on a bad form of oxygen called singlet oxygen and destroy it. A diet rich in carotenoids reduces the risk of many diseases, including cancer and age-related macular degeneration.

7. Bioflavonoids

They are also called flavonoids for short. Bioflavonoids are compounds that are derived from plants and can be divided into six groups:

1. Isoflavones (found in soy),
2. Flavonols (found in onions and broccoli),
3. Flavones (found in greens, including thyme and parsley),
4. Flavonones (found in citrus fruits),
5. Catechins (found in tea and apples),
6. Proanthocyanidins (found in grapes and cherries).

8. Minerals

Minerals such as selenium, zinc and manganese are effective forms of antioxidants. They serve as "assistants" or "helpers" for many antioxidant enzymes. The enzyme super oxide dismutase helps convert super oxide into hydrogen peroxides. The cytosolic form of this enzyme needs copper and zinc as co-factors. The mitochondrial form of super oxide dismutase needs manganese. Consuming minerals such as selenium reduces the risk of cancer. Fruits and vegetables are very high in antioxidants. Unfortunately, the food that we take everyday cannot provide the amount of antioxidants needed for cancer-fighting purposes. For example, one orange only contains about 65 mg of vitamin C. To get 2,000 mg, we will have to eat 30 oranges a day. Similarly, to get the 400 IU of vitamin E, we will have to eat almost 5,000 calories of food a day.

There is also no single antioxidant that is better than others. All of them work together hand in hand. They also serve to regenerate one another. Vitamin E's antioxidative power, for example, can be regenerated by vitamin C. Hence, they work synergistically.

SHOULD ANTIOXIDANTS BE USED?

Not too many years ago, most doctors believed that antioxidants should *not* be used because studies have shown that antioxidants protect normal as well as cancer cells against chemotherapeutic agents, rendering conventional therapy less effective.

Careful dissection of the experimental design of such studies show that cancer cells in these studies were given a single low-dose micronutrient just before the start of a series of conventional chemotherapy treatment. During the treatment, **cancer cells did show resistance to chemotherapy and radiological therapeutic agents.** It is from studies such as this that the doctors assume that all antioxidants, regardless of dosage or frequency will protect cancer cells and should therefore be avoided.

We see two flaws in extrapolating the conclusion based on this experimental design to a clinical cancer setting. Firstly, the design assumes that cancer cells react in the same way to low-dose as well as high-dose antioxidant therapy. Secondly, it assumes that only one dose of antioxidant is given. In reality, a series of doses are given during any program.

More recent studies using antioxidants in the appropriate high and repeated doses show that they **improve the effectiveness of chemotherapy and radiological therapy**. This is contrary to the conclusions drawn from earlier studies. These later studies show that antioxidants when used at high and repeated doses deter the growth of cancer cells without affecting the normal cells, a totally opposite conclusion.

Let us look further into these studies.

A single low-dose vitamin C or E micronutrient can indeed stimulate the growth of both normal and cancer cells. In a trial study on the effectiveness of beta-carotene, low doses were given to heavy smokers who actually had pre-cancerous cells in their bodies. The results showed that a single low dose of beta-carotene increases their chances of getting lung cancer. This is because both cancer and normal cells thrive in an environment of low-dose antioxidant. Smokers already have pre-cancerous cells in their body, and a low dose of antioxidant actually nurtures such pre-cancerous cells into cancerous cells.

On the other hand, in an environment of high doses of antioxidants, normal cells can protect themselves while cancer cells cannot. They will be destroyed by the antioxidants. High-dose antioxidants are therefore toxic to cancer cells but not normal cells. This is a very important lesson. Antioxidants therefore behave differently in different dosage levels. They can be an antioxidant at one dose and become a pro-oxidant at another dose. If this is not confusing enough, we now know that cells, depending on their structural health, also react differently when exposed to different levels of antioxidants.

The mechanism of action is not totally clear. It is postulated that during conventional cancer therapies, the cancer cell's defense mechanism is weakened and unable to go against the high-dose antioxidant. The supply of extra antioxidants will help the cell go through a self-repair process. Other pathways have been proposed. For example, most cancer cells lines are low in the enzyme catalayse, resulting in a buildup of hydrogen peroxide which is a pro-oxidant. Vitamin C appears to work in this pathway of increasing hydrogen peroxide load in the body if the intracellular environment of the cancer cell is high in iron (as many cancer cells are because cancer cells have a high affinity for iron). Vitamin C therefore can have both an antioxidant and pro-oxidative effect.

Most research now confirms that a **repeated high dosage of antioxidants destroys cancer cell while sparing normal cells.** In fact, many natural-oriented physicians believe that **low-dose antioxidant therapy is contra-indicated in a cancer setting.**

So far, studies have confirmed that:

- Antioxidants in low doses protect cancerous cells against the negative effects of radiotherapy and chemotherapy and should not be used.
- Different cell types have different reactions to nutrients. Melanoma cells are very sensitive to vitamin C but not so parotid carcinoma. The reverse is true for beta-carotene. The difference also depends on the nutrient dosage and the type of cancer cell.
- A single low-dose micronutrient should never ever be given before, during, or after conventional therapy as it enhances normal and cancer cell growth. Low doses of antioxidant alone can make cancer cells more active and grow rapidly. It therefore makes the situation worse.
- Some nutrients augment the effects of chemotherapy. Studies have shown that a high dose of vitamin C, beta-carotene, and vitamin E succinate causes a 50% reduction in melanoma cell growth without affecting normal cells. In other cases such as colon cancer, vitamin E has been proven to be more effective than 5FU alone in reducing metastasies.
- Antioxidants enhance the effects of hyperthermia without affecting the normal cell.

What is Therapeutic Dosage?

What should be the optimum dose of antioxidants to administer to cancer patient?

Unfortunately, there are **no standard references established yet and none is expected.** However, doctors who specialize in nutrition and natural cancer therapy will have the best idea. These therapeutic ranges have been established mainly through clinical experience.

The two terms low doses and high doses should be distinguished clearly in micronutrient therapy. Low doses are those that are established by the RDA (Recommended Dietary Allowance). They are usually given to people for prevention of diseases and for general well-being. High doses are doses prescribed to cancer patients for the purpose of destroying cancer cells without killing normal cells.

As mentioned earlier, the low and high doses for most of the micronutrients have yet to be established. In the case of vitamin C, the generally accepted daily dosage parameters are as follows:

- Prevention of scurvy – 35 mg
- Low-dose RDA – 80 mg
- For general well-being: 100 to 300 mg
- Anti-aging dose: 300 to 2,000 mg
- High dose – 2,000 to 10,000 mg
- Very high dose – for active cancer treatment and as an adjunct to conventional treatment: 5 to 50 grams
- Toxic dose – where cancer cells and normal cells are both killed: None established yet.

The amount needed varies from case to case. In general, the **dosage required to maintain cancer remission is lower than those used to treat active and growing tumors,** but will be significantly higher than those used to prevent cancer or for general well-being. In this book you will see reference to a "therapeutic dose". This is the dose that ranges from high dose to very high dose. The actual dosage used depends on the size of the patient, the kind of cancer, and the goal. Generally speaking, **dosage used during cancer in remission**

is towards the low end of the therapeutic dose range, while
active cancer treatment would require a dosage level towards
the high end of the range, if all else remains equal.

Furthermore, high-dose micronutrients should be used at least 48
hours before chemotherapy and radiotherapy to protect the normal
cells. Dietary antioxidant in high doses will enhance chemotherapy
and radiotherapy effectiveness if given in a series and on
daily basis.

SINGLE NUTRIENT OR NUTRITIONAL COCKTAIL?

Some doctors prefer to use a single micronutrient to attack cancer
cells. Others prefer a cocktail approach that uses a myriad of
micronutrients. **But most nutrition-oriented doctors seem to
favor the second approach because of the wider coverage and
lower dosage required per nutrient.**

The body needs about 50 recognized essential nutrients plus
hundreds more only found in natural whole food that is supplemented
with the proper brigade of antioxidants. The combined effect of all
these nutrients yields more than what can be have been expected
of any single nutrient. Gathering the right nutrients together at the
right time in the right ratio is the key to turn the body into an optimized
cancer-fighting machine. Nothing else comes close.

Many studies have been done to support this. A case-study was
conducted with a group of lung cancer patients who took a mixture
of antioxidants along with chemotherapy and radiation therapy. Their
intakes included 15,000 IU of vitamin A, 10,000 IU of beta-carotene,
300 IU of alpha-tocopherol, 2 grams of vitamin C and 800 mcg
(microgram) of selenium. The results showed that their survival rate
after two years was far greater than that of the control group.

Nutrients to Avoid

Beware of an antioxidant called super oxide dismutase (SOD). It should not be used in **high** dose (dosage beyond therapuetic range) together with chemotherapy and radiotherapy as it becomes dangerously resistant to oxidation.

Another group of antioxidants, namely N-acetylcysteine (NAC), tangeretin and flavonoids should also be avoided in **high** dose during chemotherapy or radiotherapy sessions. NAC reduces the effectiveness of doxorubicin, flavonoids does the sameto tamoxifen.

High dosages of any of these single nutrients are needed to elicit the above undesirable interactions. Why this interaction takes place is uncertain. Normal therapeutic doses in a nutritional cocktail have **no** side effects when taken by those in active chemotherapy or radiotherapy.

Do not take iron supplementation unless you have an iron deficiency. Cancer cells are very much attracted to iron. They also have a higher iron content compared to normal cells.

IMPORTANT CANCER ANTIOXIDANTS

We will now examine some of the common antioxidants used in cancer programs. They form part of a complete biological network consisting of over 50 different nutrients. They all function separately. Different antioxidants work on different parts of the cell. Antioxidants work as a team and no single antioxidant can function on its own. They rely very much on one another to carry out a particular function, just like one big happy family.

The following list is not complete. Also not all antioxidants are necessary for each patient. We should select the most appropriate nutrient and the right dosage based on the type of cancer and the desired goals.

1. Beta-carotene

This is a non-toxic form of vitamin A, which is otherwise a toxic nutrient if taken at too high a dose. It is a strong immunity booster, and it provides the supporting nutrients that allow the carotene to be converted into vitamin A without the toxicity. In addition, beta-carotene can also prevent free radicals from damaging a cell's DNA. Such damaged DNA can cause cancer.

Hundreds of studies have been conducted on the efficacy of beta-carotene in a cancer setting. An extensive research, for example, was carried out in Helsinki. Altogether, 36,265 people were studied to assess the relationship between the levels of vitamin A and beta-carotene. The study also examined their subsequent development of cancer. When their blood levels of vitamin A and beta-carotene were measured, those with the lowest levels had a greater risk for cancer. The report noted that cancer risk goes up when we lack these nutrients in our bodies. In another Harvard study, it was also reported that women with high breast tissue concentrations of carotenoids are less likely to have breast cancer.

Beta-carotene protects against prostate cancer in men. Japanese studies report that low levels of beta-carotene cause prostate cancer. In another study in America, it was evident that high blood levels of beta-carotene could protect the body against lung cancer, melanoma and bladder cancer. This study was performed at John Hopkins School of Hygiene and Public Health in Baltimore.

The above studies show similar results pointing to the fact that people with high intakes of beta-carotene have a reduced risk of cancer and heart disease. The reason? Beta-carotene stimulates a molecule that helps the immune system destroy cancer cells. It increases the number of receptors on white blood cells in a molecule known as major histocompatibility complex II (MHC II). MHC II is integral in helping monocytes, a type of white blood cell, direct killer T-cells to cancerous cells. In other words, beta-carotene is an important antioxidant in directing the immune system to destroy cancer cells.

Therapeutic Dosage 25,000 to 100,000 IU a day. Low-dose supplementation is not recommended, especially for smokers.

2. Vitamin C

Vitamin C is found in plants such as rose hips, apples and citrus fruits. It is a potent water-soluble antioxidant. While most animals synthesize their own vitamin C, humans do not.

Vitamin C in large doses was first used in the 1950s to prevent and treat cancer and other diseases. In 1971, Nobel laureate Linus Pauling, PhD and Ewan Cameron brought vitamin C as a cancer therapeutic modality to the forefront of medical research. Since then, a lot of attention has been paid to vitamin C and its excellent effects in cancer prevention.

The role of antioxidant in cancer prevention is now well established. Over the years, many studies have proven that people with a high dietary intake of fruits and vegetables are less likely to develop cancer. This is because fruits and vegetables contain phytochemicals and micronutrients that are antioxidants. Vitamin C is an integral part of such fruits and vegetables. The only problem is that we cannot get enough of it for its cancer fighting properties from food alone. Vitamin C, in high doses, has been shown to prevent the formation of carcinogenic nitrosamines and fecal mutagens, enhancing the immune system, accelerating detoxifying liver enzymes and blocking the toxic effects of carcinogens such as polycyclic hydrocarbons, organochlorine pesticides and heavy metals.

Animal Studies and Cell Cultures

Studies by Linus Pauling have shown that a large dietary intake of vitamin C delayed the onset of mammary tumors in mice. Vitamin C also delayed the onset of malignant dermal tumors in mice initiated by exposure to ultraviolet light.

Vitamin C and its fat-soluble derivative, ascorbyl palmitate is effective in preventing skin cancer. Vitamin C also retards colon, kidney and bladder cancer in animals. Many researchers have cited that animals treated with vitamin C had tumors that were less aggressive because the stronger cells prevented the spread of cancer.

Some in vitro studies of cell culture have reported vitamin C to be cytotoxic to several malignant melanoma cell lines, mouse sarcoma cells and mouse ascites tumor cells. At low doses, vitamin C is cytotoxic to mouse lymphocytic leukemia cells, mouse cells from a lymphoid neoplasm, human fibrosarcoma cells, and an acute lymphoblastic leukemic human cell line. Vitamin C is also cytotoxic to some non-malignant but cancerous cell lines.

Mechanisms of Action

Vitamin C is an excellent antioxidant that fights cancer. It fights cancer by:

1. Fortifying the immunity system by increasing lymphocyte production.
2. Salvaging cellular free radical damage.
3. Inhibition of hyaluronidase, keeping the ground substance around the tumor intact and preventing the spread of cancer.
4. Destroying oncogenic viruses through its enhancement of phagocytic activities.
5. Correction of an ascorbate deficiency commonly seen in cancer patients.

6. Stimulating and stabilizing collagen formation.
7. Neutralization of carcinogenic toxins.
8. Increases hydrogen peroxide and free radical generation in the cancer cell under a high iron environment.

Tumor cells are more easily destroyed when high doses of ascorbate-induced peroxidation products are introduced. This is because there is a catalase deficiency in these cells.

The Evidence

It is impossible to have a discussion about the scientific validity of vitamin C and cancer therapy without discussing the controversy stirred by the Vale of Leven and Mayo studies.

The famous Vale of Leven study was conducted by Dr Ewan Cameron and his associates, (later including Linus Pauling, PhD) at his hospital in Loch Lomondside, Scotland. This interesting study began in November 1971 with a small group of 50 cancer patients who were given a ten-day course of intravenous (IV) continuous slow-drip infusion of sodium ascorbate in half-strength Ringer's Lactate Solution. After the IV treatment, the patients were given oral doses of vitamin C of 2.5 grams every six hours for a total of 10 grams in 24 hours. The dosage varied from 10 to 30 grams daily and was continued indefinitely as long as the patient was alive. The objective was to maintain plasma ascorbate levels of at least 3 mg/dl. The researchers were happy to note an improvement in general well-being, vigor, pain relief and appetite within five to seven days. But by the 100th day of treatment, **the mortality rate was only 50% instead of the predicted 99%.** Of the remaining 25 patients, 20 died between days 110 and 659. The average survival period was 261 days. Five subjects had an average survival period of more than 610 days.

Not satisfied with the results, the doctors conducted another study in 1978 with more stringent criteria. They also improved on the design in the original study. This time around, 90% of the people who received the ascorbate lived three times longer than the control group. Long-term survival made it impossible to assess survival time with certainty for the remaining 10% of the cases. At the time the study was published, the survival rate of the ascorbate group was 20 times that of the control group. The results this time were even more promising.

In an effort to validate or refute the Cameron and Pauling results, the Mayo Clinic initiated a study on 150 advance-stage cancer patients who had previously received chemotherapy or radiation therapy. The patients were given ascorbate at the same dosage. The researchers reported no significant survival time difference between the vitamin C and placebo group. It is interesting to note, however, that the 27 patients who received no treatment lived an average of 25 days compared to an average of 51 days for the vitamin C or placebo groups. A vast majority of the subjects had received prior chemotherapy, radiation or both treatments.

Due to widespread criticism that the Mayo study had not addressed the effect of vitamin C on cancer patients who had not received prior chemotherapy or radiation, the same researchers initiated a second trial. One hundred cancer patients with advanced colorectal cancer were randomly assigned to receive either 10 grams of ascorbic acid or a placebo on a daily basis. The subjects continued on the treatment for as long as they were able to take oral medications or until there was evidence of tumor progression. When this occurred, over half of the subjects received subsequent chemotherapy (5FU) and vitamin C therapy was stopped.

The researchers did not report survival time, as they did not continue the patients on vitamin C on an indefinite basis until death. Instead, they reported that after one year, 49% of subjects who received vitamin C and 47% of the control subjects were still very much alive. Survival time was comparable to the Cameron and Pauling untreated group for both groups.

Dr Cameron and Dr Pauling disagreed with the Mayo study. They challenged it and pointed out that the study was a big mistake. What was their reason? They explain that **vitamin C cannot be started and stopped in cancer patients like a drug. The effects can only be seen with long-term therapy for life.** It does not produce immediate results like a drug, as it is not a drug in the traditional sense.

Dr Cameron says, *"You know, vitamin C is a totally different therapy that requires life long treatment and cannot be administered for just 10 weeks. Something is definitely wrong with the Mayo study."*

Uncontrolled trials conducted at two different hospitals in Japan during the 1970s also confirmed the increase in survival time of terminal cancer patients who were supplemented with ascorbate. At the Fukuoka Torikai Hospital study, the average survival time was 43 days for the 44 "terminal" patients supplemented with low levels of ascorbate (under 4 grams daily) and 246 days for 55 of the patients supplemented with higher dosages of ascorbate (greater than 5 grams daily – averaging 29 grams daily) from the time the patients were labeled "terminal".

At the Kamioka Kozan Hospital in Japan, 19 terminally-ill control patients survived an average of 48 days compared to six patients on high levels of vitamin C who lived an average of 115 days or 2.4 times longer than the control group.

While the jury is still out on the efficacy of megadose vitamin C as mainstream cancer treatment, it can still be considered as an alternative form of treatment. Today, many natural-oriented physicians use megadose intravenous vitamin C as adjunct therapies or in cases where traditional modalities have been exhausted.

Despite the unresolved debate on megadose vitamin C therapy, there is considerable epidemiological evidence pointing to the benefits of vitamin C in the prevention of cancer. Some of the following pieces of evidence are worth considering:

Bladder Cancer

An epidemiological study was carried out in Hawaii comparing 195 males and 66 females with cancer of the lower urinary tract with two matched controls. An interesting result reported was a decreased risk of cancer with an increased level of vitamin C consumption for women but not for men. Another study of 35 patients with bladder cancer showed that the serum ascorbate level was low for those with cancer.

Colorectal Cancer

Most colonic polyps develop into colorectal cancer. In a study involving 36 patients with polyps, 19 received 3 grams of ascorbate a day while 17 subjects received a placebo. The researchers noted a decrease in polyp area after nine months of treatment with ascorbate but not with the placebo. In addition, a trend towards a decrease in polyp number was found.

Stomach/Gastrointestinal Cancer

Cohen and associates examined epidemiological studies and found 9 of 10 case-control studies and 10 of 11 non-controlled studies yielded a significant inverse relationship between ascorbic acid intake and stomach cancer risk. Administration of vitamin C to patients with asymptomatic peptic ulcer resulted in a decrease in DNA damage in 28 of 43 subjects.

Safety of Vitamin C

Reported side effects of vitamin C include calcium oxalate kidney stones, B-12 destruction, iron overload, and elevated urinary uric acid. However, studies of these side effects are not conclusive especially in healthy individuals. For example, ingestion of large amounts of vitamin C results in only small increases in urinary oxalates or urates.

From a practical viewpoint, **it is prudent to avoid high doses of ascorbate in calcium oxalate stone formers, patients on dialysis or with serious kidney disease,** and possibly patients with hemochromatosis and other iron overload diseases.

There is, however, **one reported case of death associated with vitamin C intake.** In a certain sub-population of terminal cancer patients who suffered from end-stage metastasis (stage IV), the administration of high doses of ascorbate provoked tumor hemorrhage and necrosis, which resulted in the destruction of the tumor but also the concomitant death of the patient.

Intravenous Infusion

Most of us who are in good health can take up to 10 to 30 grams of ascorbate orally without any problems. But we must be careful because a high-dose vitamin C has a laxative effect. The Bowel Tolerance Level (BTL) differs from person to person. Physicians using a mega dose of vitamin C of 30 grams or more often resort to slow intravenous drip as the delivery route of choice. The most commonly used form of IV vitamin C is sodium ascorbate. The rate of infusion is kept below one gram per minute and osmolality is kept under tight control to avoid harming the veins.

While the specific protocol varies with each patient and the type of cancer involved, most IV vitamin C treatment entails a program of four weeks or more. There are two to three infusions per week, which start at a low dose of 15 grams and increase gradually. This is supplemented by oral ascorbate daily (four to 10 grams) to help prevent possible rebound effect especially on days when no infusion is given.

Vitamin C alone may not be enough of an intervention in the treatment of most active cancers. It does, however, appear to improve the quality of life and extend survival time. As such, it should be considered as part of a treatment protocol for all patients with cancer, whether they have chosen a primarily orthodox, alternative medical or complementary approach.

Therapeutic Dosage Dr Pauling recommends a dose of 1 gram to be taken 2 to 4 times a day. This amount should be gradually increased every few days by 0.5 gram until a total of 10 grams a day is reached. When you have diarrhea, you have reached the Bowel Tolerance Level (BTL). The BTL varies from patient to patient. It ranges from 4-40 grams. When diarrhea occurs, reduce the intake by 1 to 2 grams below the BTL and this will often relieve the symptoms.

In more advance cases of cancer, Dr Abram Hoffer recommends taking 12 grams of vitamin C in divided doses throughout the day. Pure crystalline vitamin C can be dissolved in either water or juice. Start with 1-2 grams a day, if there is no diarrhea, the amount of vitamin C intake can be raised by 2 grams on the following days. Mineral ascobate are preferred to avoid gastric irritation.

Your body adapts to an increasing vitamin C intake. Do so gradually at the rate of 500 mg increase every 3-5 days as tolerated. Sudden large increase may cause diarrhea. Similarly any decrease in your vitamin C intake should be done gradually. A sudden drop in vitamin C intake can lead to symptoms of scurvy such as bleeding gums during tooth brushing or easy bruising even though your actual cellular vitamin C level may be high and are well above the recommended level. It takes approximately twice as long for the body to get used to the decrease as it does to the increase. A high dose of vitamin C may also potentiate the action of vitamin E and other anti-oxidants to act as blood thinners. This may require you to lower your anti-coagulation medication or aspirin intake.

3. Vitamin E

Vitamin E is a key nutrient needed for combating the effects of cancer. It strengthens the immunity system and is an important fat-soluble antioxidant. The use of vitamin E together with chemotherapy and radiotherapy is still under study. Nevertheless, there is some reported good news.

Women with breast diseases benefit much from vitamin E therapy. This was proven in Baltimore during a study on 17 female patients and six controls. The ladies were given placebo tablets for one menstrual cycle, followed by vitamin E at 600 IUs a day for another two menstrual cycles. At the end of the study, all patients were tested for blood levels of estradiol, estriol and progesterone. The study concluded that 88% of patients reflected significant clinical improvements, confirming the fact that vitamin E is an effective treatment for breast diseases.

Vitamin E not only augments blood levels of both estriol (E3) and progesterone in fibrocystic patients, it also increases the ratio of estriol (E3) and progesterone to estradiol (E2). E3 is the natural estrogen found in the body and is anti-cancerous. Progesterone is an opposing hormone to estrogen and it counter-balances the negative effects of estrogen dominance. The latter leads to estrogen-related diseases such as breast, ovarian and uterine cancer in women.

Positive studies on vitamin E include the following:

- Highly malignant melanoma cell in vitro can be converted into normal cells after three days of exposure to vitamin E succinate.
- Glioma tumor cells, present in the brain, can be reduced by vitamin E succinate.
- Non-Hormone-sensitive cells are converted into hormone-sensitive cells when exposed to vitamin E succinate. On the other hand, hormone insensitive cells are hard to treat.
- In the case of ovarian and cervical cancer, vitamin E slow downs activities of cancer cells without affecting the normal cells.
- In radiotherapy, vitamin E succinate helps to destroy the cancer cells and protect the normal cells.
- Tamoxifen, when combined with vitamin E, is more effective in attacking breast cancer cells.

Therapeutic Dosage   d-alpha tocopherol succinate at 400 to 800 IU a day. Some doctors may recommend up to 2,000 IU a day in more severe cancer cases. Do not take the cheaper synthetic vitamin E which is far less absorbed.

4. Selenium

Selenium, a type of mineral, is a powerful antioxidant that protects cells from the bad effects of oxygen free radicals.

Certain studies have implied that selenium reduces the risk of cancer by binding with glutathione peroxidase to destroy free radicals and in so doing, protect cell membranes. Some even indicated that the use of selenium reduces bad side effects such as nausea, emesis, and headache during chemotherapy.

Intakes of 200 mcg of selenium a day has been proven to reduce cancer deaths, especially in prostate cancer. Generally, cancer patients often lack selenium in their bodies. As such, the supplementation of selenium works synergistically with vitamin E in combating cancer.

Therapeutic Dosage The intake of selenium should not exceed 500mcg a day unless under a physician's supervision. Be very careful as concentrations of selenium at 1,000 mcg or more can cause irritations of the respiratory system, rhinitis, lung edema, broncho-pneumonia and a metallic taste in the mouth. Selenium dioxide may also cause erythema and toxic necrosis of the skin, a loss of hair and nails, tooth decay or even nervous system disorders.

Conversely, high-dose zinc (more than 100 mg) supplementation should be avoided, as it is a known enemy of selenium.

5. Lipoic Acid

This is a wonderful universal antioxidant because of its ability to dissolve in both fat and water. When this acid is in a fat environment, it enhances the effectiveness of other antioxidants. Due to its soluble nature, it can cross the blood brain barrier while many other antioxidants cannot.

A major benefit of lipoic acid is that it acts as an "encourager" and helps to regenerate other antioxidants such as vitamins C and E, coenzyme Q10 (CoQ10) and glutathione. Lipoic acid can recycle vitamin E by quenching tocopherol radicals. It indirectly reduces vitamin C or increases the levels of ubiquinol (a derivative of CoQ10) and glutathione, which in turn helps to regenerate the tissue levels of vitamin E.

Therapeutic Dosage 500 to 1,000mg a day.

6. Poly-MVA

Poly-MVA is an alpha lipoic acid complex with palladium. It is a non-toxic polynucleotide reductase and has three different names, Polydox, Poly-MVA and LAPd. Here, MVA stands for minerals, vitamins and amino acids whilst LAPd stands for Lipoic acid Palladium complex.

It was discovered that platinum is very deadly to cancer cells. Unfortunately, it is also very toxic to us humans. However, its cousin palladium is not toxic to us but can act against cancers. As lipoic acid is a powerful antioxidant that is water and fat-soluble, it allows the Poly-MVA to penetrate the cell membranes and the blood brain barrier.

The primary functions of Poly-MVA are to:

• Protect cellular DNA
• Deliver the antioxidant lipoic acid into the cell
• Act as an intracellular electron donor
• Generate water within the cell

Cancer cells cannot breathe and produce little water in the cell. They use more sugar and produce no oxygen radical pathways. When synthetic DNA reductase enters these cells, protein radicals are formed and these destroy the cancer cell's proteins. Normal cells are not affected as they can convert the radicals into energy and water.

Poly-MVA also repairs cancer cells that have been abnormally altered. It improves the synergy of other nutrients while its metal components activate vitamin B-12. Additionally, it also helps to transfer energy within cells due to the lipoic acid component.

In addition to its excellent anti-cancer properties, the following benefits are also derived from Poly-MVA.

- Improving memory
- Raising energy level
- Protecting DNA from free radicals
- Chelating cadmium, mercury and lead
- Slowing the aging process and
- Increasing muscle strength.

Brain tumor patients have reported benefit from lipoic acid. High success rates have also been reported in breast, ovarian, prostate, colon and lung cancers.

In Canada, initial trials were carried out by an oncologist, the late Dr Rudy Falk. Dr Falk noted that when Poly-MVA was used in conjunction with chemotherapy, patients reported benefits such as lessened pain, improved appetite, weight gain and revitalized energy. Ten years down the road, these patients who continued to use low doses of Poly-MVA recovered completely and had no further signs of cancer.

Therapeutic Dosage Like other forms of antioxidants, the dosage level varies with patients. Those with advance cancer may take 2 teaspoons four times a day for eight weeks before tapering off. For cancer prevention, one-half to one teaspoon a day is enough. Each 8-ounce bottle contains 240 cc or 48 teaspoons of Poly-MVA. Approximately 8 to 10 bottles will be consumed the first three months. The mixture is reddish-brown in color and does not require refrigeration. So far, there are no reported side effects or associated toxicity.

Additional notes on Poly-MVA:

- Concurrent EDTA chelation therapy is not recommended because of its strong mineral content.

- As Poly-MVA needs free radicals available in the cells to transform them into energy, concurrent intake of high-dose vitamin C (more than 200 mg) is not productive. Other antioxidants such as CoQ10 are not affected.
- No additional alpha lipoic acid is needed because this is already present in the Poly-MVA and its amount is sufficient to deal with the free radicals.

7. Bioflavonoids

These compounds derived from plants are more commonly known as flavonoids. They can be divided into six groups:

- Flavonols (found in onions and broccoli),
- Flavones (found in greens, including thyme and parsley),
- Flavonones (found in citrus fruits),
- Catechins (found in tea and apples),
- Proanthocyanidins (found in grapes and cherries).

Under normal circumstances, we can obtain most of the bioflavonoids from a healthy plant based diet. There are literally thousands of flavonoids, and more are being discovered each day. For cancer fighting purposes, we will concentrate on essential ones with proven scientific studies.

A. Green tea

When this is drunk regularly during chemotherapy, tumor regression is shown. The ingredients in green tea are believed to cure cancer. But too bad, there are not enough anti-cancer components in a cup of tea. Besides, a cup also contains about 30-50 mg of caffeine, depending on how long the tea is steeped in the water. Since caffeine is a stimulant, cancer patient should best avoid green tea and take it in the form of caffeine-free extract capsules.

Therapeutic Dosage 4 to10 decaffeinated green tea extract capsules a day.

B. Quercetin

This special flavonoid destroys cancer cells whilst leaving normal cells intact. Eat more onions and apples if you want to get the best of this flavonoid.

Quercetin performs well with chemotherapy agents like tamoxifen, cisplatin, adriamycin and radio therapeutic agents. It prevents the spread of cancer by stimulating our immune system the way that the potent antioxidants reishi and maitake mushrooms do. It also alters the mitotic cell cycle and genes in tumor cells and enhances apoptosis. Quercetin also raises the intracellular glutathione level and acts well with hyperthermia treatments.

Quercetin stops mutant p53 protein. It suppresses glycolysis and ATP production, interferes with ion pump systems and various signal transduction pathways. DNA polymerase B and I are also inhibited by quercetin.

Quercetin slows down the growth of estrogen positive and estrogen negative cells. It inhibits mutant p21 genes found in more than 50% of colon cancers.

Therapeutic Dosage 2 to 6 grams per day. It is even more effective when used with vitamin C.

C. Tangeretin

This can be found mainly in citrus fruits.

Bad news was reported in a study conducted on mice. It was reported that tangeretin blocked the effect of tamoxifen in mammary cancer.

As such, do not use tangeretin in breast cancer treatment together with tamoxifen until the therapy is supported by scientific studies. In the case of low doses, it may be effective in cancer prevention.

D. Resveratrol

These are found in more than 70 species of plants, including mulberries, peanuts and particularly in grapes.

Resveratrol serves as a defensive molecule that acts against fungus in grapes and other crops. It is found in abundance in crops that are not treated with artificial fungicides. Plenty of resveratrol is found in the skin of grapes. Fresh grape skin contains about 50 to 100 micrograms of resveratrol while red wine concentrations range from 1.5 to 3 milligrams per liter.

Resveratrol is a strong antioxidant that stops the enzymes necessary for cancer growth. It also inhibits cyclo-oxygenase, a cancer promoter.

In a clinical study, cells in a HL60 human leukemia cell line that were exposed to resveratrol were destroyed. This flavonoid also prevents the development of preneoplastic lesions in mouse mammary glands treated with a carcinogen in culture. Additionally, it also inhibits other tumor growths in mice. So far, there are no reported toxic side effects.

Therapeutic Dosage 50 to 500mg per day. Cancer patients should not take alcohol due to its toxic effect on the liver.

WHAT SHOULD YOU DO?

You now know about the power of some of these proven anti-cancer antioxidants. Widespread research has proven that the careful use of antioxidants can help you combat cancer, and reduce side effects from conventional therapy if you are undergoing such a treatment.

High success rates have also been recorded in the prevention of cancer.

Through the years, occasional negative studies do surface. Such negative studies appear to be mediated by a number of conditions, including the concentration of the antioxidant, the presence of metal ions and the tumor's ability to produce antioxidant enzymes, the length of administration, difficulty of controlling parameters, and faulty experimental designs.

Generally speaking, from what we have seen clinically the past 50 years, high doses of antioxidants destroy cancer cells, while a low dose creates an antioxidant effect.

Several studies in animals have also showed that antioxidants have helped to shrink the tumor size and increase longevity. Doubtless, our knowledge of antioxidants in a cancer setting is still in its infancy stages. The interactions of antioxidant and chemotherapy cannot be predicted solely based on a set of presumed mechanisms. But luckily, more and more evidence has been gathered to prove that high and continuous doses of antioxidants are beneficial during and after chemotherapy.

Antioxidants are not the only non-toxic form of natural cancer treatment. They should be viewed in a supportive role and be combined with other drugs or conventional therapies when treating cancer. That is the best use of this class of natural therapeutic agents.

CHAPTER FIVE

OPTIMIZING
MITOCHONDRIAL FUNCTION

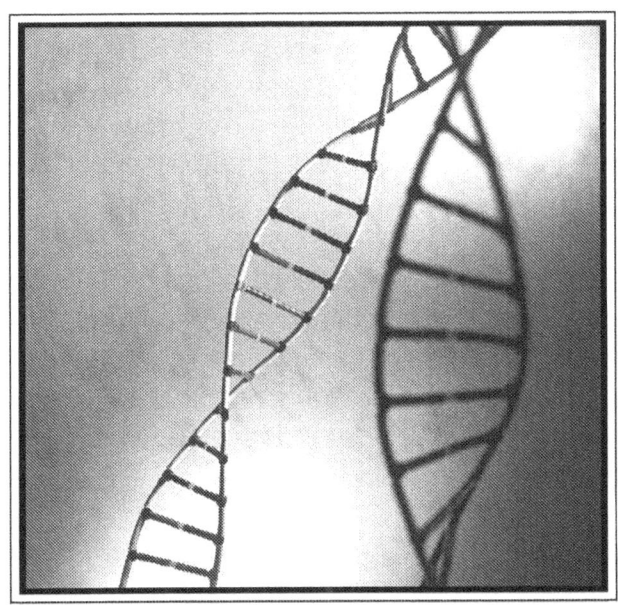

"Cancer is an energy wasting disease. Ensuring optimum
energy production is a key to cancer recovery."

*Maria Sulindro, MD, anti-aging
and physical medicine specialist.*

In the last chapter, we saw how free radicals can damage the cellular nucleus, leading to mutational changes and ultimately to cancer.

Let us now turn to the other components within the cell that can play a role in cancer-fighting as well.

Recall earlier we mentioned that cancer cells love sugar. They live on it and use it as their energy fuel, instead of oxygen. Unfortunately, this is not an effective use of resources. The amount of energy produced when sugar is used as a fuel is far less than when oxygen is used. In fact, 40% of cancer patients die of malnutrition because the food they eat is broken down into sugar which is robbed by cancer cells to the extend that regular cells are deprived of the much needed nutrition. As you will see later, one of the most important tools we have against cancer is to starve it of sugar.

Given the compromised energy generation state of our cells, are there any natural compounds that can increase the efficiency of our cell in generating more energy in our fight against cancer? You cannot fight cancer when you have no energy. Optimizing the production of energy may not be important for a healthy adult but it becomes life and death for the cancer-stricken patient.

Nutrients that are especially important to enhancing energy generation which occurs in the mitochondria include **CoQ10, magnesium, and vitamin Bs.**

COENZYME Q10

Coenzyme Q10 (CoQ10) is a benzoquinone compound made naturally in the human body. The "Q" refers to the quinone chemical group. The number "10" refers to the isoprenyl chemical subunits that are part of this compound's structure. CoQ10 is used in the body in a process called aerobic respiration, where oxygen and sugar are converted to energy.

CoQ10 enhances antibody synthesis, macrophages and T-cell activities. It prevents oxidative damages to the cell's DNA. As such, these processes help the mitochondria to generate energy. The body also uses CoQ10 as an endogenous antioxidant.

Undeniably, CoQ10 is viewed as a potent membrane stabilizer. Many scientists today believe that CoQ10 is excellent for heart disease patients. Over the past years, it has acquired a reputation for curing heart diseases. The reason is simple, cardiac cells are the most active and energy-demanding cells in the body. They keep the heart going 24 hours a day without a break. In fact, the highest concentration of mitochondria is located in cardiac cells. CoQ10 helps cancer patients by protecting their hearts from being damaged by chemotherapy drugs and effects.

Human/Clinical Studies

The use of CoQ10 as a standard conventional treatment for cancer is yet to be established. On the other hand, the good news is that in animal studies, the use of coenzyme Q10 shows good results. Inspired by this success, experiments are being conducted in various parts of the world by scientists eager to test its protective powers against the heart toxicity in cancer patients treated with the anthracycline drug doxorubicin.

A. Case-study in Denmark

In Denmark, 32 breast cancer patients were closely observed for 18 months. Their cancer had already spread to the auxiliary lymph nodes, which is not a very positive sign. What the researchers did with this group of ladies was to supplement them with vitamin C, vitamin E, beta-carotene, other vitamins and trace minerals, essential fatty acids and CoQ10 daily. At the same time, they also underwent some forms of conventional treatment.

Checks were done on these patients every three months. To help the doctors detect any signs of the cancer worsening, mammography, bone scan, X-ray or biopsy were performed. Towards the end of the study, the report showed an unbelievable survival rate of 100%! The patients also claimed that the decreased use of painkillers improved their quality of life. They also did not suffer any weight lost due to the effects of the cancer.

Out of the 32 breast cancer patients, six had warning signs that their cancer was returning. Doctors quickly gave two of them a higher dose of CoQ10. After three to four months, both patients reported complete regression of their breast tumors, confirmed by clinical examination and mammography.

B. Research Study in Texas

The first person to pioneer the study of CoQ10 was Karl Folkers, from the University of Texas.

Similar to the study in Denmark, he also chose 32 breast cancer patients, with ages ranging between 32 to 81 years. The patients are already at the advance stage as the cancers have spread to their lymph nodes. Karl Folkers instructed them to consume the following nutrients for 18 months on a daily basis in addition to their conventional treatment.

1. 2,850 mg of vitamin C
2. 2,500 IU of vitamin E
3. 90,000 IU of beta-carotene

4. 387 mcg of selenium (plus secondary vitamins and minerals)
5. 1.2 gm of gamma linolenic acid
6. 3.5 gm of omega-3 fatty acids
7. 90 mg of CoQ10

The results were quite similar to the Denmark case. Two years down the road, all the patients were still living! All 32 patients were still very much alive and kicking, although four were expected not to pull through. Six of them showed partial tumor regression.

The ambitious scientists then decided to increase the prescribed dose of CoQ10 from 90 mg to 390 mg per day in one of the patients. She was a 59-year-old woman with a family history of breast cancer and had already been diagnosed as having breast cancer. Her dosage of CoQ10 was raised to 390 mg per day. Within a month, the tumor spontaneously shrunk. After two months, mammography confirmed that her tumor had disappeared completely. Another remarkable achievement in such a short time frame! Wouldn't it be fantastic if all cancer patients can be cured in two months?

Inspired by this success, doctors decided to try this once again on another 74-year-old woman. This was a pessimistic lady who refused further surgery after learning that her breast cancer had not been eradicated by a previous surgery. She was then given daily doses of 390 mg of CoQ10. Within two to three months, clinical examination showed that her breast tumor was no longer there.

Dr Folkers explained that breast cancer patients have a much lower blood level of CoQ10 than normal people. As such, breast cancer can be suppressed by taking supplements of CoQ10. Women with low CoQ10 levels have a 38.5% chance of getting breast cancer. On a different front, cervical cancer patients have been found to have a lower level of CoQ10 and vitamin E level in their cells.

On the other hand, post-menopausal women who are on statin drugs to lower their cholesterol level have higher chances of getting breast cancer. Statin drugs, oral diabetic agents, anti-depressants, beta-blockers and hyperthyroidism will also deplete the endogenous CoQ10 levels in our bodies.

Therapeutic Dosage 100 to 300mg. Patients with concurrent heart disease will need a much higher dose of 350 to 400 mg per day. As the blood levels of CoQ10 are easily depleted in cancer patients, supplements are needed for those undergoing chemotherapy radiation therapy.

MAGNESIUM

In our bodies, thousands of enzymatic reactions take place that influence the metabolism of carbohydrates, amino acids, and nucleic acid proteins and ion transportation. 300 of these functions require magnesium which is central to the cell cycle and it is therefore an important mineral in our daily lives. It is estimated that up to 80% of the American population does not meet the RDA of 350 mg.

Magnesium controls the key rate-limiting steps in the cell cycle at the onset of DNA synthesis and mitosis which in turn control cell reproduction and growth. A deficiency of magnesium in the body reduces the efficiency of functions such as protein synthesis that are dependent on magnesium. Another function adversely affected is energy production in the cellular respiratory chain in the mitochondria. This will make the patient feel tired. A lack of magnesium also depresses cell-mediated immunity, such as phagocytic activity, as well as lymphocytic functions. Damage in the cell membrane caused by a lack of magnesium and vitamin E leads to free radicals and peroxidation of membrane lipids. These are linked to the production of cancer cells. As you can see, magnesium is vital for the continued well-being of the cell.

Hypomagnesaemia, the medical term for magnesium deficiency, is common among patients with pelvic or abdominal cancer. Significantly, some chemotherapy drugs intensify magnesium deficiency. For example, one such drug, Amphotericin B, binds magnesium to the cell membrane and makes it less active. Another drug called Cisplatin. This drug also interferes with magnesium cellular metabolism resulting in arrhythmia in which the heart beats irregularly.

Some chemotherapy drugs cause mitochondrial and nucleic magnesium depletion. This results in hemorrhage, arrhythmia and stroke. Magnesium is also depleted during radiotherapy processes, especially in the intestines where magnesium is absorbed.

Unfortunately, most people living in advance and developed countries lack magnesium in their diets. It is estimated that as much as 70% of the American adult population is not meeting the RDA of 300 mg magnesium a day. As mentioned earlier, a deficiency in magnesium can lead to cancer as immuno-competence that eliminates transformed cells, depends on magnesium. Chronic magnesium deficiency has been linked to lymphatic sarcomas and leukemia in rats. As such, optimal magnesium intake may be a prophylactic against the onset of cancer.

Interesting enough, there are some doctors who feel that magnesium supplementation has no effect on reducing tumor growth. In fact, they believe that large doses of magnesium supplementation can lead to increased tumor growth of established carcinomas.

The intake of magnesium and calcium is commonly linked. The recommended daily allowance for calcium ranges from 1,000 mg to 1,500 mg a day. In the case of magnesium, it is only 300 mg. The intake of calcium and magnesium is therefore 4:1. Some doctors said that the more appropriate dietary ratio should be closer to 1:1. Some even recommend a ratio of 1:2 in normal healthy adults.

Therapeutic Dosage Despite controversial findings that magnesium deficiency might be implicated in the treatment of cancer, we should maintain a **calcium/magnesium ratio of 1:1 for those with cancer.** Magnesium supplementation of about 500 to 750mg a day is recommended.

B COMPLEX VITAMINS

Vitamin B complex performs a variety of functions. One of the important functions is to produce energy at the cellular level. If you have a well-balanced diet, you should have enough B vitamins. However, cancer patients may require supplements for optimum body function.

Therapeutic Dosage Vitamins B1, B2, B3, B5, and B6 should be taken in optimal dosage. Cancer patients may benefit from a higher dose of B3 and B5. They also often lack vitamin B12 due to their absorption problems. But, a word of caution, high doses of vitamin B12 may lead to cancer instead. Therefore, oral or sublingual doses of vitamin B12 should not exceed 3,000 mcg daily or 1,000 mcg intramuscularly (that is by injection) twice a week. Niacinamide 1,000 mg - 1,500 mg as well as panthothenic acid 900 mg - 1,500 mg is also recommended.

CHAPTER SIX

BOOSTING YOUR IMMUNITY

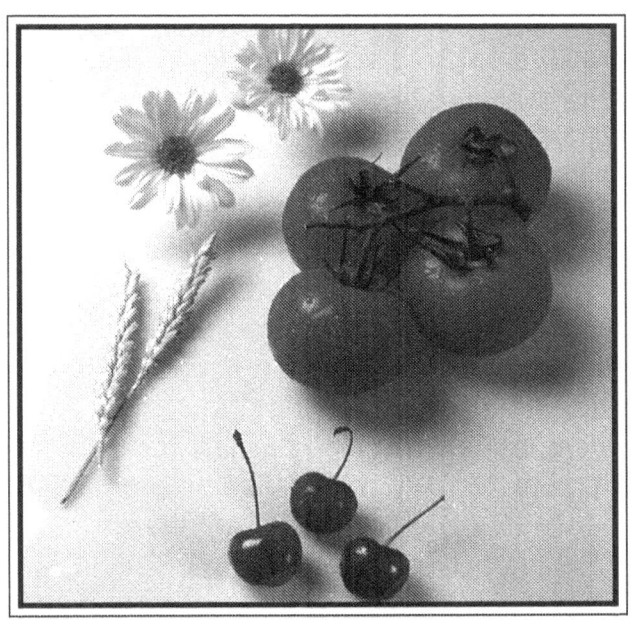

"If you don't address the immune system,
you're treating cancer without really treating
the cause of cancer."

Victor A Marcial-Vega, MD, Radiation Oncologist in
The Definitive Guide to Cancer

> *At least 95% of all cancer patients are immuno-suppressed due to physical, chemical, mental, and/or environmental causes.*
>
> — Marcial-Vega, MD, radiation oncologist and alternative cancer physician.

O ur body fights bacteria and germs via a magnificent and well coordinated network of cells, organs and glands. This defense network is called our immunity or natural defense system.

This defense army consists of a whole team of soldiers. They use different weapons such as the lymph system, sweating, fevers, excretion, phagocytes, white blood cells, lymphocytes, white blood cells and immunoglobulins. They all work together to protect the body from external and internal insults.

Maintaining a well-balanced immune system lays the foundation to good health and longevity. Today, we all know that the immune system plays an important role in preventing and fighting cancer. More and more cancer researchers now pinpoint a weak immune system as a primary causative factor in cancer. Addressing the immune system is therefore a key to any comprehensive cancer treatment program, conventional or otherwise.

BASICS OF THE IMMUNE SYSTEM

The soldiers of our immune system are called antibodies. There are many different forms of antibodies. They are classified into five major classes, IgA (immunoglobulin A), IgD, IgG, IgM and IgE. Each class has its own function. They work together to ensure that all foreign bodies are destroyed.

In our immune system are two important elements called T- and B-lymphocytes. B-lymphocytes make and distribute antibodies in our bodies. T-lymphocytes are in charge of the cell's immunity. They act as a command post from which most orders for the immune system flows. They stimulate macrophages and B-lymphocytes. T-lymphocytes are the pillars for protecting the body from diseases such as bacterial infections, strong viruses, fungi, cancer, and parasitic infections.

T-lymphocytes are assisted by a group of T-helper cells. They help to control various white blood cells by issuing chemical codes known as cytokines. Some examples are interleukins and interferons. T-helper cells coordinate the actions of white blood cells and destroy unwanted substances.

Our bodies also manufacture T-suppressor cells to slow down the destructive activities of cytokines from other white blood cells. This is an important function as it serves to protect the healthy cells. The correct ratio of T-helper to T-suppressor cells is crucial. It maintains a balance between the aggressive actions to destroy bad cells whilst protecting the good cells.

According to alternative physician Douglas Brodie, MD, HMD physician who is licensed both in homeopathy and allopathy,

> *Many patients tend to believe that if they get rid of a tumor, then have succeeded and nothing more needs to be done. However, it is precisely at this point that diet and supplements play their most profound role, helping to keep cancer from recurring.*

Today, biology's greatest achievements have given us much research findings about the immunity boosting agents derived from natural sources. Scientists have so far pinpointed many as immunity-building agents. We will now look at a few examples, how they originate, their effectiveness and their usage.

1. Cat's Claw

Cat's claw is also called "una de gato" in Spanish. It can be found on trees in the rain forests of the Andes Mountains, particularly in Peru. It is a 100-foot long woody vine.

This herb has been investigated at many centers in Peru, Austria, Germany, England, Hungary and Italy since the 1970's. These studies have concluded that the herb is useful in the treatment of arthritis, bursitis, allergies, diabetes, chronic fatigue syndrome, cancer, herpes, organic depression, menstrual irregularities and disorders of the stomach and intestines.

Compared with Echinacea, golden seal, astragalus, and Siberian ginseng, cat's claw is far superior in its antibacterial and immune building properties.

Cat's claw enhances the immune system in a general way. The unique alkaloids found in cat's claw enables white blood cells to better swallow and digest harmful organisms in the body. The most immunologically active alkaloid is called isoteropodine or isomer A. Cat's claw has been proven to increase the production of leukocytes and T4-lymphocytes, thus blocking the advances of many viral diseases.

Also, the excellent antioxidant properties of cat's claw help prevent the hardening of the arteries and heart disease. Long ago, way beyond the time of our forefathers, the bark of the root was used as the medicinal part. Today, the bark from the vine is used.

Therapeutic Dosage One cup of infusion to be drank three times a day or 1 to 2 ml twice a day. In the form of dry standardized extract, 20 to 60 mg is to be taken daily. The amount should be increased to

2 to 6 grams a day for those in remission and tripled in advance-stage cases.

As cat's claw may cause the immune system to reject foreign cells, anyone with an organ or tissue transplant should not take it. If you are suffering from auto-immune illnesses, multiple sclerosis or tuberculosis, you should also avoid it. Cat's claw is not suitable for pregnant women and children below two years old. Those people on blood thinners such as aspirin or warfarin should use it carefully with a physician's guidance as it may also block platelets from forming blood clots and increase the effectiveness of blood thinning drugs.

2. Olive Leaf

This is a relative newcomer in the antioxidant arena. It only made its maiden appearance in the mid-1980s. Despite its being a relatively new discovery in America, successful studies have indicated that it can treat illnesses caused by certain retroviruses, bacteria or protozoans. Influenza, the common cold, meningitis, Epstein-Barr virus (EBV), encephalitis, herpes I and II, human herpes viruses 6 and 7, shingles, HIV/ARC/AIDS, chronic fatigue, hepatitis B, pneumonia, tuberculosis, gonorrhea, malaria, dengue fever, bacteremia, severe diarrhea, blood poisoning, and ear, urinary tract and surgical infection can also be treated with olive leaf extract.

Some people have claimed the benefits of olive leaf such as relief for psoriasis, normalization of heart beat irregularities and less pain from hemorrhoids, toothaches and chronically achy joints.

The active ingredient in olive leaf is called Oleuropein. It is made from an ingredient found on olive trees that protect the trees against insects and bacteria.

Research and extensive medical studies confirm that olive leaf extract is anti-viral because it can damage the harmful viruses and bacteria in an infected person. It also has other healing properties such as:

1. An ability to interfere with amino acid production for viruses;
2. An ability to contain viral infection and spread by preventing virus shredding, budding or assembly at the cell membrane;
3. The ability to directly penetrate infected cells and stop viral replication.

Olive leaf extract can boost our immune system by increasing phagocytes in white blood cells. This leads to a destruction of foreign bacteria and viruses that are literally gobbled up by the phagocytes.

Therapeutic Dosage The standardized extract is the best. It contains at least 20% of active ingredients. The recommended dosage is 500 mg to 2,000 mg a day.

3. Essiac Herbs

This herb has the most interesting origin. Long ago, in Canada, the Ojibwa native tribe's medicine men had a mixture of herbs to treat illnesses. Later, in 1922, this formula was passed on to a Canadian nurse called Rene Caisse. She asked for this formula as a standby in case she ever needed it in future.

One day, her aunt fell ill with cancer and was given six months to live. Left with no other alternative, Rene decided to try out this tea on her dying aunt. A miracle happened. Her aunt survived and lived on for another 21 years. She eventually died of old age. This tea was then named "Essiac" spelling Rene's family name backwards.

Inspired by her aunt's success with the tea, Rene Caisse began to offer this wonderful and magical recipe to anyone who asked for it. Soon thereafter, Dr Charles Brusch, who was the doctor to former US President John F. Kennedy, learned about the success story of the tea. He became very interested and became a research partner with Rene.

Nurse Caisse mixed four different herbs, namely burdock root, slippery elm, sheep sorrel and turkey rhubarb root. The different herbs work together harmoniously to purify the blood, help cell repair and ease pain.

Burdock Root (67.7%)

This herb shows promise for helping to slow down cell changes and stop cancer. It prevents gall and kidney stones. It contains vitamin A and selenium, which helps to eliminate free radicals. The burdock root also contains chromium, which is useful in regulating blood sugar.

In another two experiments conducted at the National Cancer Institute, one showed that burdock root had anti-tumor activity in animal tumor systems. The other reported no significant activity. Later, in another study, this same organization, claimed that when the substance benzaldehyde was isolated from burdock, the results showed anti-tumor activity in the animal tests. We can see from the conflicting results that additional studies are needed.

Slippery Elm (5%)

This herb is rich in calcium, magnesium, vitamins A, B, C, and K. When eaten, it can soothe organs, tissues and mucus membranes. Not only is it effective for those with lung problem, it can also aid digestion and relieve asthma.

Slippery elm dissolves excess mucous in organs, tissues, lymph glands, and nerve channels, and eases wastes through the alimentary canal. When tested at the National Cancer Institute, it showed no anti-tumor activity in mouse leukemia systems.

Slippery elm also contains beta-sitosterol and a polysaccharide, both of which have been reported to have anti-tumor activity in animal tumor studies.

Sheep Sorrel (21.6%)

This herb was heralded as a potent remedy for cancer some decades ago. It was used to relieve internal ulcers, clear skin problems such as eczema, ringworm and herpes. Being richly endowed in minerals, vitamins and trace elements, it helps to nourish the glandular system in our bodies.

When aloe emodin is removed from sorrel, the latter manifests significant anti-leukemic activity. Dr Chester Stock at Sloan-Kettering in New York remarks, *"The Sheep sorrel can help to destroy cancer cells in our bodies."* He came to this conclusion after conducting some successful experiments. When a similar test was done at The National Cancer Institute, it was reported that no activity was found in mouse leukemia systems.

Turkey Rhubarb Root (5%)

This herb acts as a gentle laxative and purges the body of wastes and toxins. It helps digestion. It also contains a substance called rhein that controls bacteria in the intestines.

In the test of animal sarcoma-37 systems, anti-tumor activity was demonstrated. On the other hand, at the National Cancer Institute, two samples were tested and found to have no anti-tumor activity in mouse leukemia systems. Clearly there is much contradiction and controversy among these findings on the herbs and their anti-cancer functions.

Essiac Tea has been used for over 80 years, with good anecdotal reports for treating cancer, AIDS, diabetes, inflammatory skin problems, liver ailments, influenza, fevers, inflammation, thyroid disorders, stomach ulcers and other old-age diseases.

Studies have revealed that this blend of tea breaks down nodular masses to normal tissues. This helps to ease pain. Some patients say that their tumors are enlarged and hardened after a few treatments. But, fortunately, they start to soften later. Sometimes, pus is also discharged from the infected areas.

Strengthening the immune system is the main objective of Essiac tea. Nurse Caisse has said that even if the tumor does not disappear, its potency and invasive character is reduced. She recommends the herbs be used for six to eight treatments before surgery. After that, it should be taken once a week for at least three months.

It is obvious that our knowledge of how Essiac works is limited at best. As Dr Hoffer, MD, PhD, author of *Vitamin C and Cancer*, puts it, *"I'm not sure what Essiac does to extend cancer survival, and for all we know it may not have this effect. On the other hand, it's not toxic and my patients have reported feeling good while taking it, so why not support them?"*

Common sense tells us that the most effective treatment comes from **brewing the tea from raw herbs** bought from reliable herbalists. You should follow strictly the instructions for preparing the tea. Many people may find this method a bother and too time-consuming. Such being the case, they take either an extract or the essence of the tea. Some busy people may choose to drink the tea that has been bottled. In fact today, most of the tea come in commercially preparations. These are ideal for general preventive measures but not for cancer treatment due to their low potency. Some companies have produced these herbs in a capsule form but we are not sure about the efficacy of such crushed herbs. The most effective form is still the raw herb or the essence extract.

A word of caution: Over the past few years, researchers have tried to improve the blend with additional ingredients, including other herbs and medicinal mushrooms. Already several popular commercial versions of this tea have added other herbs to the original four herbs. Be very careful. For example, herbs such as red clover have also been included in some concoctions. Due to its hormone-like effect, it is not certain whether people with hormone-sensitive tumors such as breast cancers should consume such "improved" versions of the tea.

Here is a recipe for making essiac tea from raw herbs.

The Essiac formula :

> 6 cups of Burdock Root (cut)
> 16 ounces of Sheep Sorrel herb (powder)
> 1 ounce of Turkey Rhubarb Root (powder)
> 4 ounces of Slippery Elm Bark (powder)

Preparation:

1. Measure out 8 ounces of the Essiac mix (the dry formula above).
2. Place two gallons of distilled water in a stainless steel kettle.
3. Bring the water to a brisk boil (about 30 minutes).
4. Put Essiac dry mix into the boiling water, stir and boil hard for about 10 minutes.
5. Allow to sit and cool slowly for six hours.

6. After six hours, stir it thoroughly with a wooden or stainless steel ladle.
7. Let it sit for another six hours.
8. Return kettle to stove and bring to a boil again.
9. When the boiling point is reached, turn off the heat and pour the contents through a stainless steel strainer into a second stainless steel kettle.
10. Clean the first kettle thoroughly.
11. Strain the contents a second time from kettle two to kettle one.
12. Pour the herbal tea immediately into dark amber bottles and seal them while still hot. (Note: Dark amber bottles may be purchased from most any drug store or pharmacy.)
13. Store in refrigerator.

Therapeutic Dosage This varies from 1 to 2 oz a week to three times a day. **Don't take too much,** for this can be dangerous. The most commonly recommended daily dose is 2 oz or 4 tablespoon diluted in 2 to 3 oz of water. This is to be taken once a day for the first 10 days, after which, the dosage shall be reduced to 1 oz in the same dilution per day. The maximum dose is 6 oz daily in 2 to 3 divided doses for advance cases. It should be taken for a minimum period of one to two years or even longer if necessary. As the cancer improves, the dose can be reduced to two or three times per week. Heat 2 oz (four tablespoons) distilled water, then mix it with 2 oz of Essiac tea taken directly from the refrigerator. Essiac tea should be taken at bedtime on an empty stomach, at least two hours after eating. It can be taken in the morning on an empty stomach. If taken in the morning, do not eat for at least two hours after taking it. Keep the Essiac tea refrigerated at all times. Shake well each time before pouring.

Essiac tea is most effective when it is brewed from the original herbs that have been organically grown. It can be combined with other anti-cancer treatments.

This tea is absolutely prohibited for people with bowel obstructions. (Note that while the tea helps to improve transit time, if bowel is already obstructed, taking the tea can lead to bowel perforation.) Avoid drinking the tea also if you have kidney disease, ulcers and colitis. Lactating and pregnant women as well as children below 12 years of age should not take this tea either. People on anticoagulant therapy must consult an informed doctor when taking the tea.

4. Hoxsey Herbs

Up till today, the Hoxsey herbs are regarded as the biggest hoax in America's medical field. Just like many cures in natural medicine, this label has not been entirely justified.

Way back in 1900, Harry Hoxsey invented this herbal formula for treating cancer. It consists of two remedies, one to be used externally, the other internally.

The external mixture consists of a red paste containing antimony trisulfide, zinc chloride, bloodroot, and a yellow powder containing arsenic sulfide, sulfur, and talc. This mixture is believed to destroy cancer cells. The internal mixture is a liquid containing licorice, red clover, burdock root, stillingia root, barberry, cascara, prickly ash bark, buckthorn bark and potassium iodide. This mixture is for immune boosting. The mixture can be applied directly on the skin or drunk as a tonic. When taking the Hoxsey herbs, patients are to avoid pork, vinegar, tomatoes, carbonated drinks and alcohol. Instead, they are encouraged to use immune stimulants, yeast tablets, vitamin C, calcium, laxatives, and antiseptic washes as well as to think positively.

However, many doctors were dead against Hoxsey and strongly criticized his ideas. Despite his successes, the American Medical Association labels this treatment the worst cancer quackery of the century.

Hoxsey's idea is to stimulate the body's immune system to overcome cancer. By supplying the body with herbs together with digestive enzymes, iodine and potassium compound, Hoxsey herbs provide the necessary nutrition. The herbal remedies can strengthen the immune system

Horxey's herbs contain a high concentration of potassium iodide. While iodine itself does not have significant anti-cancer properties, it helps the thyroid gland to function properly. At the same time, potassium helps in cells metabolism.

The thyroid gland regulates the temperature in our bodies. People with under-active thyroids have a lower body temperature. As cancer cells cannot stand heat, we have to maintain a slightly higher basal body temperature to create an environment unfavorable for cancer growth.

Therapeutic Dosage   This depends on your specific needs and whether the cancer is internal or on the skin surface. Be careful, some of the ingredients in the Hoxsey formula have negative side effects. Buckthorn bark may give you nausea and diarrhea if taken in large doses. Cascara, too, can cause diarrhea. When barberry root is given to rabbits, it causes swelling of the kidney and cardiotoxicity.

5. Fish Oil

Fish and its oil, once mocked by doctors as useless remedies are now fulfilling claims beyond folk medicine's wildest dreams by emerging as one of the most potent dietary supplements. Fish oil contains a high dose of omega-3 fatty acids that helps to protect the body against a long string of diseases.

Fish oil stops the spread of cancer and stops the formation of new blood vessels as well. It counterbalances the effects of omega-6 fatty acid's production of inflammatory econsinoids. This is because omega-3 and omega-6 fatty acids compete for cell receptors in the cell membrane. Omega-6 fatty acids also produce prostaglandin E2. This causes a weaker immune system, suppression of cytokines, attenuation of T-cell proliferation, inhibit macrophages and natural killer cells responsible for cancer growth.

Furthermore, omega-6 fatty acids support the formation of new blood vessels (angiogenesis) in many cancers and therefore helps cancer cell growth. Conversely, fish oil prevents cancer cells from being attached to healthy tissues. It also slows down the rate of tumor attachment in the lymph nodes. It is used as a useful adjunct during chemotherapy and radiotherapy as well. Fish oil enhances cytotoxicity of chemotherapy drugs, including mitomycin, cisplatin, and vincristine. Experiments with low doses of fish oil fed to mice protected them from methotrexate-induced small intestine damage. Human studies also confirm that fish oil increases the efficacy of chemotherapy drugs. Breast cancer patients with high fat tissue levels of omega-3 fatty acids respond better to chemotherapy. In short, omega-3 prevents cancer from spreading with or without chemotherapy.

Therapeutic Dosage Most high potency fish oil provides 1,000 to 1,500 mg of fish oil with about 300 to 500 mg of EPA and 200 to 300 mg of DHA per capsule. About 6 to 9 capsules are needed daily in advance cancers. Fish oil in large doses has a blood-thinning effect. People who are on blood thinning medicine such as coumadin should not consume excessive amounts of fish oil.

6. Iscador

Iscador is a fermented preparation of the European mistletoe which is a semi-parasitic plant that grows on deciduous trees. Found in many areas of Europe, America and Korea, it is used to treat cancer.

Long ago, iscador was hailed as a potent medicine in the treatment of serious illnesses. We now know that it stimulates the immune system. In 1920, it began to be used for treating cancer. Today, iscador is given to patients in two ways. The first is as a central component of a complex treatment regimen. In the second, it is given to patients as a single agent. Iscador is now recognized in Germany and Switzerland as a medicine. It is also used widely throughout Europe at holistic clinics.

Rats with cancer showed a 78% reduction in their thymus gland when given iscador. The thymus gland is a central component of the immune system. Studies have shown that iscador reduces tumor size and prolong lives. Patients with cancers of the cervix, ovaries, breast, stomach, colon, and lung should try using this herb. It can also cure cancers of the bone marrow, connective tissue, lymphomas, sarcomas, and leukemias.

Therapeutic Dosage   Iscador is given by injection, near the site of the tumor or directly into the tumor. Direct tumor injection is most common for tumors of the liver, esophagus and cervix. A treatment course can last from several months to many years. The injections are given early in the morning three to seven times a week. The entire course consists of 10-16 injections given in increasing concentration and adjusted depending on the patient's general condition, sex, age and the type of cancer.

Most of the time, there are hardly any side effects. But once in a while, allergy symptoms, higher body temperature and flu-like symptoms are reported. Sometimes, the injection site is inflamed and abdominal pain with nausea may occur.

The berries in the mistletoe may look beautiful but are actually very poisonous. Keep them out of reach of babies and children. If accidentally taken, you might have seizures. Also, people on antidepressant drugs should not take this herb. When taking this herb, you must be very careful and use it under close supervision of your doctor. Do not self-medicate with this herb.

7. Medicinal Mushrooms

There are altogether 100,000 types of mushrooms. About 700 types can be eaten; another 50 types are poisonous whilst another 50 have medicinal effects. Some mushrooms are very pretty but almost all medicinal mushrooms look tough and woody. We can never judge a mushroom by its appearance.

Research on the use of mushrooms in treating cancer began in the 1970s. Today, scientists have confirmed their unique healing properties and have made it known that mushrooms enhance the immune function and the work of the T-cells.

The three types of anti-cancer drugs extracted from mushrooms are Lentinan derived from shitake; Schizophyllan derived from suehirotake, and PSK derived from kawaratake. These mushrooms have anti-cancerous effects because they contain a polysaccharide compound called beta-glucan. Beta-glucan has been found to exhibit potent anti-tumor activity in numerous animal studies.

A. Maitake Mushroom

This Japanese mushroom is nickname "hen of the woods," as it grows in clusters that resemble the tail feathers of a hen. Animal studies have extensively analyzed this mushroom's effect on cancer cells. When the dried mushroom powder was mixed into the animal's food, it could control and stop cancer.

Like all other mushrooms, maitake's action is that of a host defense potentiator. However, it reigns over the rest of the mushrooms in the inhibition of tumor cells. The beta-glucan present in the mushroom activates the natural killer cells of our immune system. Japanese mushroom specialist, Dr Hiroki Nanba says that the optimum dose is 25 mg per kg of body weight. He also suggests the dose to be increased by three to four times when it is used as a supplement to conventional treatments.

He discovered that four different fractions make up this special mushroom and called them Fractions A, B, C and D.

When maitake D fraction is used with half the dose of chemotherapy, it shows tremendous effectiveness in stopping cancer growth. In Japanese studies, prolonged survival rates were reported when maitake was used together with chemotherapy. The D fraction is also very effective when taken by mouth to enhance the natural killer cell, IL1. It has an advantage over beta-glucan as the latter is only effective through injection.

In another study, D fraction prevents breast cancer by 80% when given orally. When given during the early stages, the growth of the cancer cell is cut down by 70%. The recurrence rate using maitake power is 20% but for the D-fraction, it is only 10%.

Maitake extract kills cancer cells in prostate and breast cancers. In liver cancer, a combination of maitake D fraction when taken during chemotherapy at half dose shows good results. An amazing 96% success rate has been reported. However, when D fraction is taken alone, the percentage falls to 75%. In the case of mitomycin C, the percentage is only a pathetic 46%.

Therapeutic Dosage Take 30 to 100 drops of Maitake Pro-D fraction and 2 to 8 grams of whole mushroom powder a day. Exercise caution when buying maitake mushroom powder as there are many forms of it in the market. Always look for the genuine ones. Also be careful not to take too much as mushroom powder contains fiber that is hard to digest. You may get a stomach upset. Take the extract form of maitake mushroom instead. In the market, many suppliers do not disclose the extraction ratio. However, do note that a 100 mg of 8:1 extract is the same as taking 800 mg of dry powder. The higher the extraction ratio, the less you have to take and you will still get the same good results. Good quality extracts run from a 4:1 to 8:1 extraction ratio. However, they are usually more expensive than the powder form. But spending this amount of money may be worth your while in the long run.

Maitake extracts when taken with 2,000 mg of vitamin C is even more effective. Some breast and prostate cancer patients reported a lowered prostate marker called PSA (a marker for prostate cancer) after taking this combination. Not much is known about the side effects of maitake. In rare cases, allergies have been reported but not to a significant extent. Today, maitake mushroom is served as a delicious dish in many high-class restaurants. You can also buy them from the common grocery stores.

B. Reishi Mushroom

This pretty mushroom has a dark and shiny reddish-orange cap. However, a pretty surface doesn't always tell the inside story.

In ancient days, the Chinese and Japanese used this mushroom to treat liver disorders, hypertension and arthritis. It is ranked by the Chinese as one of the most potent medicinal plants in nature.

Reishi has proven anti-allergic, anti-inflammatory, anti-viral, antibacterial, and antioxidant properties. In vitro experiments show that reishi can help fight tumors. A protein, which is isolated from reishi called Ling Zhi-8 can reduce the risk of transplant rejections.

Reishi is hard, bitter and difficult to swallow. You can consume it either as a brew or ground in capsule form. Reishi has been proven to protect the liver, as a tonic for the heart and central nervous system, to lower cholesterol, and prevent allergic responsiveness. It can also increase the production of Interleukin-1 and 2 and stop tumor growth.

Like in maitake mushroom, the active anti-cancer compound is also beta-D-glucan. Beta-D-glucan is made up of a huge sugar molecule. Within this molecule are little sugar molecules chained together to bind amino acids. These sugars stimulate the immune system by activating immune cells such as macrophage and helper T-cells. They also increase the antibodies' effectiveness in producing a better response to bad cells.

According to Japanese scientist Dr Fukumi Morishige, reishi performs a better function when combined with high doses of vitamin C. The polysaccharides in the reishi are big molecules that are difficult to absorb, but vitamin C helps to break them down into smaller molecules called oligoglucan. The body can easily absorb these. As such, vitamin C increases the bioavailability of reishi and enhances its anti-cancer effects.

The benefits of reishi are wide. Besides treating cancer, it is also good for the relief of arthritis, menopausal anxiety, asthma, hypertension, hypothyroids, insomnia and heart disease.

Therapeutic Dosage   Take 150 to 900 mg of concentrated reishi extract daily. Dr Morishige recommends a larger dosage from 2 to 10 grams for cancer patients. The standardized extracts give the best results. These are usually more expensive but they are genuine and up to the mark.

C. Shitake Mushroom

The commonest edible and best-studied mushroom with the greatest proven therapeutic powers is the shitake mushroom. We can buy these mushrooms in Asian markets or your local health food stores. This type of mushroom has lots of meat. They taste delicious and are often served as a dish or as an ingredient in a variety of dishes at home or in restaurants. Its use originated during the Ming Dynasty in 1368 A.D. During that period, it was esteemed as a longevity tonic.

Shitake contains cortinelin, which is a strong antibacterial agent. It also produces an extract containing lentinan which stimulates the production of T-lymphocytes and natural killer cells. Modern studies confirm that shiitake can cure cancers and treat AIDS. In this mushroom there is a substance called eritadenine that helps body tissues absorb cholesterol and lower the amount circulating in the blood.

Japanese scientists back in 1969 conducted an animal study and isolated a polysaccharide compound from shiitake called lentinan as mentioned above. When lentinan was given to mice with cancer, their tumors disappeared in an amazing 80 to 100% of the subjects. They concluded that lentinan is able to boost immune-system cells in clearing the body of tumor cells.

Therapeutic Dosage Take 2 to 6 grams daily in standardized extract.

D. Agaricus Blazei Murill (ABM)

About 30 years ago, two curious researchers from Penn State University set forth on a journey to a village called Piedade. They discovered that the natives were happy-go-lucky, very fit and had very low rates of disease. They lived in a bed of roses and enjoyed longevity. To find out their secret recipe, the researchers launched an investigation and discovered that these natives favored eating a mushroom called Agricus Blazei Murill (ABM).

The two men found that the polysaccharide contained in this mushroom spurs production of interferon and interleukin. This effect destroys and prevents the spread of cancer cells. Later, they also discovered that ABM could cure Ehrlich's ascites carcinoma, sigmoid colonic cancer, ovarian cancer, breast cancer, lung cancer, and liver cancer as well as other solid cancers. In experiments performed on mice injected with cancer-causing agent Sarcoma 180, the injection of ABM was found to be effective in curing 90% of these animals.

Therapeutic Dosage 2 to 6 grams a day or its equivalent in standardized extract form.

E. Cordycep Sinensis (CS)

This is a rare and precious tonic found on the high plateaus of southwestern China at 3,000-4,000 meters above sea level. It is also called caterpillar fungus and comes in the form of a fine light beige powder. In Chinese, Cordycep means "summer plant, winter worm". They grow by infecting insect larvae with spores that germinate before the cocoon is formed. The fruiting body of the Cordycep grows from the dead host.

This tonic promotes phagocytosis of peritoneal macrophages, enhances the function of the reticuloendothelial system and reduces cholesterol levels.

The ancient Chinese swore by this herb. For more than 1,000 years, it has been used to strengthen their health and enhancing their immunity after a bout of chronic illness. It is also used to treat lung disease, impotence and restore renal functions. Cordysep is excellent for boosting cardiovascular health. Taking this herb can also help you to stay young and energetic.

It is ideal for convalescing patients. It helps to boost appetite, enhance blood functions, and cure respiratory tract problems and susceptibility to colds or flu.

In China, this herb is reputed for successfully treating cancer patients. The reported effective success rate is an astonishing 78 to 94.2%. The same percentage of success is also reported in other illnesses such as bronchitis, heart diseases, leukemia, lung diseases, cirrhosis, B hepatitis, and diabetes.

Therapeutic Dosage   Take 1 to 3 grams a day. Upmarket cordysep is very expensive and can cost over $1,000 per pound. Today, cordycep cultured through bioengineering processes has significantly lowered the cost.

Take the standardized extract of 2:1 extract ratio that contains at least 20% of the active ingredient, beta-glucan. A capsule of this strength will yield about 140 mg of polysaccharide. The normal dose is 1 to 2 tablets per day. In more serious illnesses, the dosage should be increased by two or three folds.

Summary of Medicinal Mushroom

Medical mushrooms are well-known for immunity boosting. Centuries ago, people began using it as a tonic and folk medicine for curing diseases.

Today, scientists are conducting much research and experiments on mushrooms. It is very clear that each mushroom has its own unique anti-cancer properties. **Maitake, reishi, shitake, and agaricus are good choices for anti-tumor activity. Cordycep is often used as a strengthening tonic for convalescing patients.**

In today's commercial world, enterprising mushroom vendors will try to promote their own as the most effective. Their prices also vary. The consumer should be cautious and only buy from reputable and reliable suppliers.

Medicinal mushrooms have a high content of fiber. Be careful not to eat too much of it, as it may be difficult for the digestive system.

8. Ukrain

The first clues of the medicinal value of ukrain came in 1978. An Austrian scientist by the name of Dr Wassyl J. Nowicky discovered ukrain by marrying two components. One is a herb called Greater Celandine. The other is a cytotoxic drug called Thiotepa.

Greater celandine is a poppy-like plant that is full of juice. It has a long and outstanding folk history of disease-fighting successes. This plant contains alkaloids such as chelidonine that has anti-cancer potential.

The marriage of this herb and drug has given birth to the compound ukrain that is non-toxic to normal cells. This new product has the ability to destroy cancer cells.

Pregnant hamsters and rats showed no signs of toxicity in their embryos when this compound was injected into them. The only side effect was a slight decrease in the average hamster litter size. In another study conducted with healthy human volunteers from Poland, Austria, and Germany, those who received repeated courses of the new drug had little side effects. Some local pain was reported in a few cases but it was not significant. Others informed that they felt a little drowsy, thirsty and had to go to the toilet more often.

Ukrain was found to activate an enhanced immune system mechanism so that the body can destroy the cancer. It prevents the development of new blood vessels needed for cancer growth. The cancer cell is starved and unable to grow. Ukrain can also cure leukemias, lung cancer, colon cancer, central nervous system cancer, melanoma, ovarian cancer and renal cancer.

In another study, Ukrain was given intramuscularly or intravenously every day or every second to fifth day for a period of ten days to three months. A slight pain was reported during intramuscular injection in the weaker patients. It was found to be effective for treating early-stage cancers. The success rate is high in the early-stage cancers and is drastically lower in advance cases.

Ukrain is primarily available in holistic clinics in Europe and Mexico.

9. Lactoferrin

This is a natural component from the milk of cows and humans. Lactoferrin helps to build immunity and maintains a stable amount of good bacteria in the intestines. As such, the number of bad bacteria like *E. coli* and *streptococci* are controlled. Lactoferrin inhibits several viruses that cause HIV and herpes. Its anti-cancer function is quite unique as cancer cells contain more iron than normal cells. Lactoferrin helps to bind iron in the cell and blood. It is able to do this because it has a strong attraction for iron. This is very important in later-stage cancers where metastasis is of primary concern.

Therapeutic Dosage 300 mg to 1,000 a day in divided dosages.

10. Inositol Hexaphosphate (IP-6)

Inositol hexaphosphate or IP-6 is derived from natural sources such as corn, grains, and legumes. People from Finland, whose diet is rich in IP-6, have a lower incidence of colon cancer.

IP-6 increases the activity of the cancer suppressor gene called p53 by as much as 17 times in some studies. The latter is responsible for inhibiting the pathway normal cells take they when turn into cancer cells.

IP-6 can help in a wide variety of cancers. A larger dose is required for solid cancers compared to blood-based cancers such as leukemia. Successful studies revealed that when IP-6 was added to liver cancer cells, the cancer cells stopped spreading. In animal studies, when liver cancer cells were injected into mice, 71% of the mice had cancer. When liver cancer cells pretreated with IP-6 were injected, believe it or not, no sign of cancer emerged.

Prof AbulKalam M. Shamsuddin, the world's leading professor of pathology at the University of Maryland School of Medicine in Baltimore said, *"IP-6 can slow down or stop the growth of liver cancer cells in mice. It does not kill cancer cells. Instead, it converts cancer cells and makes them behave like normal cells."* To reinforce his point, he added, *"Another compound called inositol can prevent colon cancer in animals. Inositol, by itself is less effective than IP-6 alone. But, when you put the two together, the effects are synergistic."*

In addition to its anti-cancer function, IP-6 can help lower cholesterol levels, thus reducing the risk of heart disease and stroke. It also prevents diabetes and kidney stones.

Therapeutic Dosage The recommended dose for cancer prevention is 1,000 to 4,000 mg a day. This should be taken in two to three divided doses. Active cancer patients need to take 5,000 to 10,000 mg a day in divided doses before food. IP-6 is very safe even at extremely high doses.

ADDITIONAL FACTORS TO BOOST IMMUNITY

A. Immunity-lowering drugs such as glucocorticoids prescribed for asthma and other inflammatory conditions should be avoided.

B. Get sufficient sleep and rest. They are very important.

C. You should have a proper routine of exercise daily to build up your immunity.

D. Live a less stressful lifestyle. You may need a drastic change if your present life is too pressurizing. Reducing stress will normalize the adrenal gland and reduce production of internal cortisol, an anti-inflammatory and pro-aging hormone.

E. Cut down on all forms of alcohol which is toxic to the liver.

F. Start a proper diet and nutrition regimen. Supplement with your diet with vitamins A, C, E, B6 and folic acid. Moderate supplementation with zinc, chromium, magnesium and selenium is also recommended.

G. Take more immune boosting supplements such as resveratrol, amino acid arginine and glutamines. Herbs such as Echinacea, goldenseal and glandulars such as thymus extract can help to support a normal lymphocyte proliferation and maintain a healthy immune system.

CHAPTER SEVEN

STOPPING CANCER SPREAD

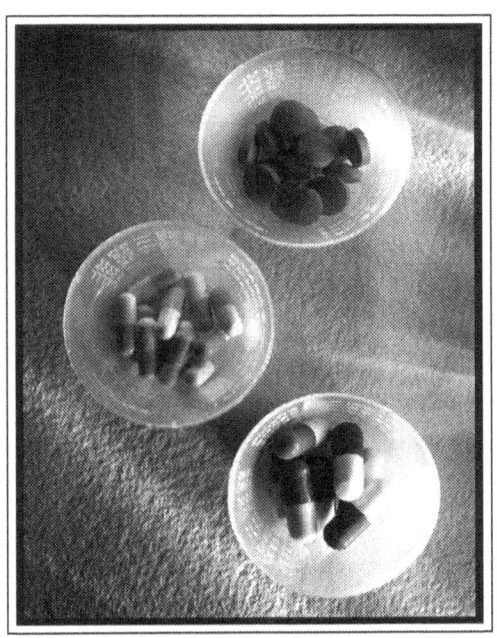

"I employ vitamin C as a first line
of defense against cancer."

Cardiologist and natural medicine pioneer Dr Robert Atkins, MD in
Dr Atkins' Vita-Nutrient Solution

C ancer can spread like wildfire. They can quickly cause much irreparable damage to our bodies. To extinguish this fire, we must first understand the ideal conditions for cancer to spread. It is now known that in order for cancers to spread to other parts of the body, they must be able to live in the following locations in our body:

1. The "home turf" of epithelial tissues where the primary organ of the cancer resides.
2. The connective tissues that surround the primary organ.
3. The tissues of a distant organ site.

HOW DOES CANCER GROW?

Cancer cells grow and develop in three phases.

Phase 1 – Initiation
When a free radical or carcinogen changes the genetic make up of a cell, the cell divides more often than it normally does. This is the beginning stage.

Phase 2 – Promotion
In this phase, the damaged cell multiplies uncontrollably.

Phase 3 – Progression
In this phase, **cancer grows through the process of invading the surrounding tissues and forming new blood vessels.** It does so by releasing compounds that go against the body's natural defense and penetrating into the surrounding tissues. The cancer cell builds itself a blood supply network through angiogenesis and invades surrounding tissues. **Without sufficient blood vessel supply, solid tumor growths cannot grow bigger than 1-2 mm in diameter.**

Certain natural compounds have been shown to retard the spread of cancer cells in any combination of the above three phases.

These natural elements include calcium D-glucarate, curcumin, resveratrol, milk thistle, shark cartilage, bovine cartilage, vitamin C, L-proline, L-lysine, and bindweed. We will now look at their properties, functions and effectiveness in preventing the spread of cancer.

ESSENTIAL NATURAL COMPOUNDS TO STOP CANCER SPREAD

1. Calcium D-Glucarate

D-glucaric acid is a non-toxic natural compound that contains a beta-glucuronidase inhibitor. This "stopper" possesses the ability to enhance detoxification of carcinogens and tumor promoters by stopping beta-glucuronidase and preventing hydrolysis of their glucuronides in the liver.

In a study conducted, calcium D-glucarate was compared with a chemotherapy drug called 4-HPR. The results were monitored based on the first two phases of cancer and showed that calcium D-glucarate reduced tumor multiplicity. The percentage was the lowest at 28% for stage I and the highest for stage III at 63%. The study also reported two more points:

1. For patients in their second and third phases of cancer, the gloomy news is that calcium D-glucarate is not effective in preventing cancer spread at these stages.

2. Chemo-preventive effect was synergistic when calcium D-glucarate was used together with 4-HPR.

Therapeutic Dosage 100 to 200 mg a day.

2. Curcumin

Curcumin is a carotenoid pigment extracted from turmeric. It helps to inhibit the progression of colon and skin cancers caused by chemicals. At the same time, it can also prevent adenoma multiplication and growth.

Colon cancer patients may be pleased to note that curcumin works best in the promotion phase (phase 2). Studies have revealed that cancer cells exposed to curcumin show shrinkage, chromatin condensation, DNA fragmentation and programmed cell death in human kidney and liver carcinomas.

Curcumin stops the formation of new blood vessels as well (phase 3). In addition to its anti-cancer properties, it is also a potent antioxidant. Curcumin also inhibits abnormal platelet aggregation that can lead to a heart attack or stroke.

Therapeutic Dosage   1,000 to 5,000 mg a day in divided dosage.

3. Milk Thistle

This compound should be introduced to all liver cancer patients. Milk thistle contains a special extract called silymarin. This herb acts as an antioxidant, protects the liver from damage and enhances the detoxification process. **It is far superior to vitamin C and E in its effectiveness.**

Silymarin helps to protect the liver from toxic chemicals such as carbon tetrachloride, amanita toxin, galactosamine and praseodymium nitrate. It also prevents the depletion of glutathione that is essential for detoxifying harmful chemicals in the liver.

Silymarin has been shown in experiments to increase the level of glutathione by 35% more. In human studies, silymarin plays a significant role in treating liver diseases of various kinds including cirrhosis, chronic hepatitis, fatty infiltration and inflammation of the bile duct.

Therapeutic Dosage 70 to 200 mg, one to three times a day.

4. Resveratrol

As discussed in the earlier chapter, Resveratrol (pronounced as rez-VER-a-trawl) is one of a group of natural compounds called phytoalexins that are produced in plants.

Resveratrol is effective against cancers at all three phases of their growth. Its anti-carcinogenic properties are a result of its conversion to piceatannol. When resveratrol is metabolized in the body by the cytochrome P450 enzyme, it creates a metabolite called piceatannol. This is an anti-leukaemic agent.

This is how resveratrol can inhibit all three phases of cancer.

1. Inducing quinone reductase activity. This is an enzyme that can detoxify carcinogens in phase 2 cancers. It can detoxify carcinogens, thereby destroying them.

2. Inhibiting cyclo-oxygenase. This is a substance that induces the production of prostaglandins. The latter stimulates tumor growth, suppresses the immune system and activates carcinogens. In this way resveratrol controls cancers in phases 1 and 2.

Therapeutic Dosage 50 to 500 mg a day.

5. Powdered Shark Cartilage

Cancers grow and multiply via the development of new blood vessels in phase 3. This process is called angiogenesis as explained earlier on.

Cartilage is a tough and elastic connective tissue. There is no blood supply in cartilage as it contains many anti-angiogenic substances.

Shark cartilage is a good example. Long ago, people often wondered why the sharks in the ocean seldom develop cancer. They were very much intrigued and their curiosity led scientists to embark on various studies into it. Experiments were conducted based on the notion that the shark's body must contain anti-cancer agents. But, which part? The shark is so big. They later found out that it was in the cartilage. Of course, today, we know that present generation sharks do develop cancer. This may be due to the changing environment. Nevertheless, shark cartilage has proven to be a rich source of an anti-angiogenesis agent. It can stop vascular endothelial growth factor. This factor stimulates human umbilical endothelial cells in culture that sometimes result in cancer.

Since then, the use of shark cartilage has created a lot of controversy and stirred up many emotions. Still, there is no conclusive evidence that it inhibits angiogenesis in patients with cancer.

Therapeutic Dosage It is very important to note that shark cartilage **only works in recommended high doses.** The recommended dosage is 0.5 to 1 gram per kg of body weight. It is quite a large dose to be taken.

To see its full effects, shark cartilage should be consumed for two to four months. Many people have difficulties taking this amount as it results in nausea. At this high level, the high calcium content in shark cartilage may aggravate hypercalcemia, which is a serious side effect of cancer. Other side effects include nausea, vomiting, abdominal cramps, constipation, hypertension, and hyperglycemia.

6. Liquid Shark Cartilage

This is an alternative to the powder form. A 7-cc vial is the same as 60 to 80 grams of shark cartilage powder. We can get liquid shark cartilage in both frozen and non-frozen forms but the frozen form is reported to be more potent.

Liquid cartilage prevents the formation of capillaries in a fibrin matrix culture. It also increases vascular permeability of the skin and the pancreas.

In treating cancer, lower doses are required for the first two phases. Do not use liquid cartilage for two to three weeks before surgery and six to eight weeks after surgery so as to allow time for the wounds to heal. Heart disease patients, please avoid this shark cartilage in any form. Children, pregnant women, nursing mothers, body builders or competitive athletes must also stay clear of them. Some reported side effects are nausea and vomiting.

Shark cartilage is not the same as bovine cartilage. While both have anti-cancer and anti-angiogenic effects, **bovine cartilage primarily acts as an immune booster although it has some angiostatic properties.**

7. Bovine Tracheal Cartilage (BTC)

The origin of bovine tracheal cartilage (BTC) dates back to the early 1950s. Many people have been using it to treat conditions including cancers, tumors and arthritis ever since.

It is a non-toxic material and has demonstrated anti-mitotic, anti-angiogenic and anti-inflammatory activities. It was developed by the aspiring and ambitious Dr John Prudden. He noted that all his subjects recorded remarkable remissions in pancreatic cancer, breast cancer, and glioblastoma multiforme during a study. The reported success rate was 90%. Another 61% had complete remission. Such encouraging results! In this study, both oral and injected forms were used but the oral form was found to be more effective.

The quest to prove the effectiveness of this cartilage has continued. In 1994, another group of doctors conducted a similar study. Using BTC as a supplement in 35 patients with metastatic renal cell carcinoma, it was reported that within three months, 22 of the patients had no relapse of the disease. There were also two patients in stable condition.

This bovine cartilage functions in immune modulation through its polysaccharide components. When these are taken orally, they can be an immunity boosting and anti-tumor agent. These polysaccharides are also present in maitake mushroom.

Therapeutic Dosage 3 to 5 grams daily in powder form in capsules. Take them before meals. This cartilage is much cheaper than shark cartilage. For cancer patients, the requirement may be more at 9 grams a day. We can only see the benefits of this cartilage after a few months. Some reported side effects are gastric upset, fatigue, nausea, fever, dizziness, and edema of the scrotum.

8. Bindweed

Earth is full of this weed. Every farmer pretty much regards it as a pest. They damage precious crops such as corn and wheat by wrapping themselves around the plants and strangling them.

They are sometimes called "the cancer of crops" as they are so much dreaded and feared – just like cancer in human beings.

Much as it is hated by farmers, laboratory studies have shown that the proteoglycan mixture found in bindweed is 100 times more effective than shark cartilage by weight. Studies in Kansas have shown that proteoglycan mixture inhibits angiogenesis in chicken egg chorioallantoic membrane tests.

So, the nuisance weed has medicinal value and it seems we can never judge something by its outward properties. Bindweed may be a killer to plants but for mankind, it can save lives.

In addition to its angiogenesis inhibiting properties, it is also a moderate immune stimulator. Studies performed on this weed's effect on human lymphocyte growth in vitro have reported an increase in lymphocyte production from 35 to 46%.

Therapeutic Dosage 1,000 to 3,000 mg per day. Raw bindweed is poisonous. However, the poison is removed during the extraction process. We should only take the standardized extract form of this weed.

9. Collagen-Matrix Reinforcement

Cancer cells spread when the nucleus secretes special enzymes. These special enzymes eat their way into the surrounding tissues, thus allowing the cancer cells to penetrate them easily. With the enzyme, cancer cells force their way into smaller vessels. They eat their way through the lumen of the blood vessel and enter the main blood stream. The blood then transports these cancer cells to distant organs. This is how secondary tumors commonly occur.

Collagen is the extracellular structure that the cancer cell must invade when spreading. The more collagen-digesting enzymes produced by the cancer cells, the faster secondary tumors are formed. A strong matrix will prevent the advance of cancer cells by resisting the digestive power of these enzymes.

We must therefore maintain a strong extracellular collagen matrix to prevent the spread of cancer cells. There are three important nutrients that help to maintain collagen, namely vitamin C (in the form of ascorbic acid, mineral ascorbates and ascorbyl palmitate), L-lysine, and L-proline.

A. Vitamin C

Apart from its properties as a strong antioxidant, vitamin C also **helps to build a stronger extracellular matrix**. This strong collagen matric will protect the healthy cells and guard against the spread of cancer cells. As our bodies cannot manufacture vitamin C, supplementation is essential for maintaining our body's collagen.

Collagen is replaced by chemical "bridges". These chemical bridges are formed by "OH groups". They help to anchor amino acids lysine and proline molecules in collagen. In the process, vitamin C is actually destroyed and used. The more collagen we wish to form, the more vitamin C has to be available.

We can see that vitamin C is an important foundation of natural cancer therapy. Ascorbyl palmitate should be used as a supplement in conjunction with vitamin C (ascorbic acid). The former is a fat-soluble form that can be retained in the body much longer than its water-soluble counterpart. Its potency is therefore many times higher than simple vitamin C. Since large doses of vitamin C are normally needed, some people may develop gastric irritation. Taking vitamin C in the form of mineral ascorbates will often bypass this problem.

In the words of Dr Linus Pauling, the father of vitamin C therapy and two time Nobel laureate,

If the megavitamin treatment were to be started at the time of first diagnosis of cancer, as an adjunct to appropriate conventional therapy, the cancer death rate could be reduced by 25% of its present value, and moreover, if in the course of time, a reasonable megavitamin regimen were to be followed regularly by every person, as a way of improving health and decreasing the incidence of cancer and other diseases, the cancer death rate would fall to one eighth of its present value.

Therapeutic Dosage 3-15 grams a day for the collagen building purpose.

B. L-Lysine

This is an amino acid that our body cannot produce. It is vital for forming collagen fibers and works together with vitamin C to form a strong collagen extracellular matrix to prevent cancer cells from spreading. L-Lysine is supplied through either our diet or from dietary supplements.

Therapeutic Dosage 2-5 grams a day.

C. L-Proline

L-Proline is another amino acid that is also an important component of collagen. Our bodies can produce L-proline but the amount is limited. Cancer patients will deplete their bodies' production in no time. Supplementation is required to ensure that the collagen matrix is strong and not easily penetrated by the collagen-digesting enzymes.

Therapeutic Dosage 1-2 grams a day.

10. Artemisinin (Wormwood) – From Malaria to Cancer

Many marvels of modern medicine are discovered by accident. Some of these include: -

1. The discovery of penicillin by Alexander Fleming.
2. The use of saw palmetto to prevent benign prostate enlargement.
3. Digoxin to enhance cardiac function.
4. Gingko to reduce vascular viscosity and increase blood flow.

Recently, another ancient herb called artemisinin was discovered. History documentation showed that it was used to treat intestinal parasitic infections, hemorrhoids (its an anti-inflammatory) and malaria as early as 2000 years ago.

The Use for Malaria

This treatment for malaria was, however, lost over time. It was only rediscovered in an archeological dig in the 1970s where its medicinal use was found in a recipe inside a tomb. The formula was dated back to 168 B.C. where the Chinese chemist isolated the primary active ingredient from the leafy portion of plant called A. annua L.

In 1972, scientists in the West called this crystalline compound "qinghaosu" or "artemisinin". Since then, studies in China and Vietnam have confirmed that artemisinin is a highly effective compound with close to 100 percent response rate for treating malaria. It has the ability to destroy the malaria parasite by releasing high doses of free radicals that attack the cell membrane of the parasite in the presence of high iron concentration. In fact, over one million malaria patients have been cured via this method. Their symptoms also subsided in a matter of days.

However, the treatment using this herb to treat malaria is not approved for use in the U.S.A due to the concern that it has a 21 percent recrudescent rate. Scientists believe that this is more likely due to patients not taking the compound for a long period. Many of them actually stop taking it as soon as their symptoms subside.

Artemisinin comes in a few derivatives, including the oil soluble artemether, which has been found to induce neurotoxic symptoms in animals in high dose (but not reported in humans). For those who are technically inclined, the activities of all artemisinin derivatives are dependent on their internal endoperoxide bridge. It is therefore a close relative of hydrogen peroxide therapy. While the exact mechanism is still under intense research, it has been shown that this herb works via highly reactive oxygen-based free radicals that becomes activated in the presence of iron. Iron is an oxidant, and our body tries to protect us from excessive iron moving it to a binded state such as hemoglobin and enzymes. The malaria parasite accumulates iron by infecting iron-rich red blood cell. Excessive iron that is spilled onto the surrounding tissues will activate the artemisinin to generate a burst of free radicals that attack the iron rich cells, killing the parasite in the process.

In other words, this compound works well in an iron rich environment (remember that malaria lives in the red blood cell rich in iron) through the release of free radicals that serve to damage the malaria organism. It is also interesting to note that drugs known to work by enhancing oxygen radical effects such as doxorubicin can enhance the effects of artemisinin.

For malaria, there is no resistance nor toxicity at the dosage of 3 grams, (about 50mg/kg) administered over a 3 to 5 day period. It is especially useful in the treatment of drug resistant malaria.

Outside of the United States, artemisinin is the number one natural herb used for malaria treatment.

The Use for Cancer

So far, the most extensive study on the use of Artemisinin as an anti-cancer agent was carried out by bioengineering scientists Drs Narenda Singh and Henry Lai of the University of Washington. This study was reported in the Journal Life Science (70 (2001): 49-56).

Iron is required for cell division, and it is well known that many cancer cell types selectively accumulate iron for this purpose. Most cancers have large number of iron attracting transferring receptors on their cell surface compared to normal cells. In laboratory studies of radiation, resistant breast cancer cells that has high propensity for accumulating iron revealed that artemisinin has 75 percent cancer cell killing properties in a 8 hours and almost 100 percent killing properties within 24 hours when these cancer cells are "pre-loaded" with iron after incubation with holotransferrin. On the other hand, the normal cells remained virtually unharmed. Another study showing the effectiveness of artesunate in treatment of cancer was also published in Oncology (April 2001: 18(4): 767-73).

The fact that iron content of cancer cells is high has also been used in another anti-cancer therapy called Zoetron therapy, where iron containing cancer cells are induced into motion using a magnetic device to induce resonance. Resonance generate heat. Cancer cells are more sensitive to heat compared to normal healthy cells. When cancer cells are heated to a certain temperature, they die while normal cells still survive.

Artemisinin is effective against a wide variety of cancers as shown in a series of successful experiments. The most effective is leukemia and colon cancer. Intermediate activities were also shown against melanoma, breast, ovarian, prostate, CNS and renal cancer. Although artemisinin is insoluble in water, it is able to cross the blood brain barrier (the water soluble artesunate is the weakness among the derivates) and may be particularly suitable for curing brain tumors, together with Poly-MVA (an metalo-vitamin)

In laboratory studies, iron needs to be added to enhance the effects of artemisinin. Within the human body, no such addition is necessary, as iron already exist in the body. It can also be taken orally and therefore high doses are not required. Some people believe that as nitrogen (tertiary amine) is absent in ART, cancer cells cannot get rid of it once it enters into the cancer cell. As a result, ART stays in the cell much longer.

In addition to the high affinity for iron in aggressive cancer cell types, most cancer cells also lack the enzyme catalayse and gutathione peroxidase. Catalayse breaks down hydrogen peroxide. A low catalayse content means a higher hydrogen peroxide load, which can release superoxide free radicals when properly stimulated to do so. This is in fact one common mechanism among chemotherapeutic agents as well as vitamin C. These traits make cancer cells more susceptible to oxidative damage as compare to normal cells in the presences of hydrogen peroxide. For this reason, concurrent administration of vitamin C in high dose is suggested.

According to Dr Rowen, a naturally oriented medical doctor and editor of the medical newsletter " *Second Opinion*" , the Hoang family of physicians in Vietnam had used arteminisin in the treatment of cancer for years. They have reported that, over a 10-year period, more than 400 patients were treated with artemisinin in conjunction with a comprehensive anti-cancer program with 50 to 60 percent long-term remission rate. The safety record of artemisinin has well been studied for over 25 years. No significant toxicity in short-term use for malaria at high dose of up to 70 mg/kg per day has been reported.

Artemisinin is not a stand-alone chemotherapeutic agent. A combination of nutritional supplements (such as green tea, CoQ10 and pancreatic enzyme) as well as a good anti-cancer diet is required.

ART may be administered orally, with a 32 percent bioavailability as compared to injections. It is highly bound to membranes. Laboratory measurement of its serum level is therefore not exact.

Forms of Artesminin

There are three common forms of artemsinin. The water soluble form is called artesunate . It is the most active and the least toxic. It also has the shortest life within the body Artemether is the lipid soluble form. It has the longest life but also the most toxic in high dosage that is seldom needed. The biggest advantage of artemether is that it can cross the blood brain barrier. Artemisinin is the active parent compound of the plant. It's half-life is intermediate. It is also very safe, and can cross the blood-brain barrier. Some clinicians prefer to use a combination of all three forms, while others tend to favor the use of artemisinin alone with great success.

Toxicity and Side Effects

High doses of artemisinin can produce neurotoxicity such as gait disturbances, loss of spinal and pain response, respiratory depression, and ultimately cardiopulmonary arrest in large animals.

In human beings, there are very few reports of adverse effects except for one case of first-degree heart block. According to Robert Rowen, MD, there is a dose related decrease in reticulocyte count for 4 days after artesunate or artemether at doses of 4 mg/kg per day for 3 days. However, the count returns to normal by day 14. When artemisinin suppositories are used, doses as high as 40 mg/kg per day have no effects on the reticulocyte count. In a study, it was reported that up to 35 percent of the volunteers had some form of transient drug induced fever.

When ART is tested with monkeys, they showed no toxicity when they received up to 292 mg/kg of artemether over 1 to 3 months. This is equal to a human dose of 20,000 mg for a 70 kg male (Journal of Traditional Chinese Medicine 2(1):31-36 1982). In another study, there was also no sign of toxicity in over 4000 patients. This does not exclude possible cases of long-term cumulative toxicity which is unknown at this time.

Cautions

A. No artesminin should be taken within 30 days of radiation therapy because of possible free iron leaks to the surrounding tissues after radiation therapy.

B. Preliminary laboratory studies include: CBC, reticulocyte count, liver function test, ferritin, TIBC, ESR, C reactive protein, and appropriate tumor markers. If the iron load is low, supplementing iron for a few days can be considered prior to starting artemisinin.

C. Tumor markers may increase during the initial stages as the tumor starts breaking down.

D. Vitamin E may work against the effectiveness of ART in vitro. However, this has not been shown to be a concern in human clinical cases.

Dosage

The therapeutic dose ranges from 200 mg a day (for cancer in remission) up to 1,000 a day (in divided doses 4 times a day) for those with active cancer. Some doctors are recommending up to 1,600 mg per day based on a 100 pounds, 5 feet 2 inches tall female.

Artemisinin should always be taken with food. Cod liver oil may be administered at the same time to enhance absorption. Generally,

400 to 800 mg per day can be used for at least 6 to 12 months. After that, it can be tapered off slowly.

Artemisinin is a "cooling herb" in the traditional Chinese medicine perspective, and some may find it too "cooling" with symptoms such as tingling. If this occurs, then the dosage should be reduced.

Despite its seemingly high degree of effectiveness, it is important to note that artemisinin is not a stand-alone compound. Concurrent use of high dose pancreatic enzymes, daily enema, liver detoxification, and periodic laboratory measurement should also be considered as part of an overall aggressive anti-cancer program.

Product Concerns

Due to the increasing popularity of this product, the consumer should exercise extreme caution and buy only from the most reputable supplier. Only genuine and pure artemisinin should be used, and only buy from sources you are familiar with.

Since the herb comes from China and South-east Asia, proper quality assurance on purity and standardization is of tremendous importance. High-grade artemisinin must always be confirmed by independent laboratory analysis on a batch-by-batch basis to ensure consistence and purity.

CHAPTER EIGHT

BALANCED INTERNAL TERRAIN

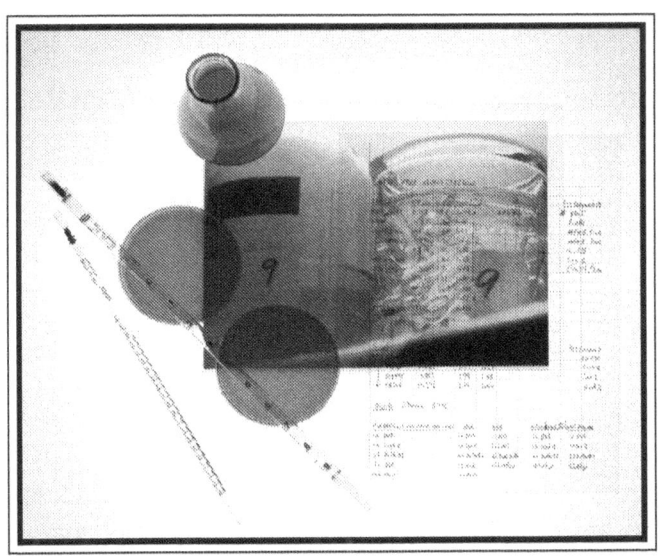

"The microbe is nothing, the terrain is everything."

Louis Pasteur, Father of Modern Pathology.

Our internal biological terrain determines the environment in which cancer cells exist. The two components of an optimum terrain are a balanced acid/base environment and balanced intestinal flora.

An acidic environment helps cancer to grow, while an alkaline environment deters cancer growth. This terrain is also influenced by the amount of friendly or unfriendly bacteria present and the transit time for food passing through the gut. Clearly we must maintain a strong and healthy biological terrain to prevent the growth of cancer cells.

Let us examine these two main components in more detail:

ACIDITY – ALKALINITY (PH)

According to the research of Dr Enderlein, our bodies can only be healed of any chronic illness when our blood is at a normal, or slightly alkaline pH.

What exactly does pH mean? pH is the short form for potential hydrogen. The pH of any solution is the measure of its hydrogen-ion concentration. The higher the pH reading, the more alkaline and oxygen-rich the fluid is. The lower the pH reading, the more acidic and oxygen-deprived the fluid is. The pH ranges from 0 to 14, with 7.0 being neutral. Indications above 7.0 are alkaline and below 7.0 are considered acidic.

The pH indicators are an exponent number of 10. A small difference in pH will translate to a big difference in the number of oxygen or OH-ions. **A difference of 1 in a pH value means ten times the difference in the number of OH-ions**. A difference of 2 means one hundred times the difference in the number of OH-ions.

In other words, a blood with a pH value of 7.45 contains 64.9% more oxygen than blood with a pH value of 7.30.

Our blood pH has a very narrow range of around 7.35 to 7.45. If our body's pH deviates from this range, we will be sick or have symptoms of falling sick. If our blood pH falls below 6.8 or above 7.8, our body cells will stop functioning and death will occur. Only when the pH level is balanced can our bodies effectively assimilate vitamins, minerals and food supplements. As such, our body's pH determines good health.

What then happens when the body is too acidic? An acidic environment will:

1. Decrease the body's ability to absorb minerals and other nutrients.
2. Decrease energy production in the cells.
3. Decrease the body's ability to repair damaged cells.
4. Decrease the body's ability to detoxify heavy metals.
5. Enable tumor cells to thrive.
6. Make the body more susceptible to fatigue and illness.

Two main factors leading to cancer are an acidic pH and a lack of oxygen. As such, are we able to manipulate these two factors so as to prevent and control cancer?

The vast majority of terminal cancer patients have a very acidic pH. Research has proven that terminal cancer patients often have an acidity level 1,000 times more than normal healthy people. Why is this so?

The reason is simple. Without oxygen, glucose undergoing fermentation becomes lactic acid. this causes the pH of the cell to drop. In more advance cancer cases, the pH level can even fall lover to 6.0 or lower. The basic truth is that our bodies simply cannot fight diseases if our pH is not properly balanced.

The normal human cell is slightly alkaline and has an abundance of molecular oxygen. The cancer cell is acidic and cannot survive in an oxygen rich environment.

How to Test Your pH Level

1. Salivary pH Test

Just wet a piece of litmus paper with your saliva 2 hours after a meal and match it against the color scale. This will give you a reflection of your state of health. Although saliva is generally more acidic than blood, it is a fairly good indicator of health. It tells you what your body retains. Salivary pH is a fair indicator of health for extracellular fluids and their alkaline mineral reserves.

The optimal pH for saliva is between 6.4 to 6.8. A reading lower than 6.4 means that there is not enough alkaline reserves. After meals, the saliva pH should rise to 7.8 or higher. If there is no increase, it will imply that the body has a deficiency in alkaline minerals especially calcium and magnesium. Food will not be absorbed and assimilated well. To deviate from an ideal salivary pH for an extended time will lead to illnesses.

If the salivary pH level remains too low, we should take more fruits, vegetables and mineral water and avoid strong acidifiers such as sodas, whole wheat and red meat to maintain its balance.

2. Urinary pH Test

The pH of the urine is an indication of how well the body is working to maintain a proper pH of the blood. It reflects the efforts of the body via the kidneys, adrenals, lungs and gonads through the buffer salts and hormones. The urine also shows the alkaline building (anabolic) and acid tearing down (catabolic) cycles. By taking urine samples, we can get a fairly accurate picture of our body pH as our kidneys filter out the buffer salts of pH regulation. The same litmus test can provide blood pH estimates based on what the body is eliminating. The urine pH can vary from around 4.5 to 9.0, but the **ideal range is still 5.8 to 6.8.**

To increase the alkalinity in our blood, we can consume these foods: almonds, aloe vera, apples, apricots, bee pollen, buckwheat, cabbage, cantaloupe, celery, carrots, cucumbers, dates, pulse, figs, grapefruit, honey, lettuce, millet, parsley, raisins, peaches, pineapple, soy products, sprouted seeds, cooked spinach, turnip tops, wakame miso soup, azuki beans and mineral water.

INTESTINAL FLORA

Do you know that good gastrointestinal health is possible only when good and bad bacteria are in balance? Both types of bacteria are needed for normal bowel functions; an efficient digestive system can prevent carcinogenic toxins from building up.

Probiotics are good bacteria. Many scientists believe that diseases are caused by toxin secretion from pathogens and not the pathogens themselves. Today, this hypothesis has been proven true. Toxins from infectious bacteria, fungi and viruses cause cancer. For example, human *papilloma* virus causes cervical cancer, *H. pylori* causes stomach cancer, hepatitis causes liver cancer and HIV virus leads to Kaposi sarcoma. In the case of some liver cancers, the secretion responsible is called aflatoxin, found in peanuts.

On the other hand, approximately 400 types of good bacteria live in the intestines. Their total population is about 100 times more than the number of cells in our bodies. Their numbers are huge but they live together in harmony. They act like security guards by guarding the intestines and preventing bad bacteria and fungi from getting out of hand. Such good bacteria help to keep our bodies healthy and fit.

When enemies attack, this ideal environment is disrupted. Then, bad bacteria, parasites and fungi such as *clostridia*, *salmonella*, *staphylococcus*, *blastocystis hominis* and *candida albicans* will proliferate in the intestines. They will start to multiply and attack the good bacteria. War is therefore inevitable.

Apart from the good bacteria's ability to guard our bodies from enemies, they also produce vitamins such as biotin, folic acid, niacin, pantothenic acid, riboflavin, thiamin, vitamins B6, B12 and K. These bacteria help to break down proteins into amino acids. Amino acids are then reconfigured into new proteins that are useful for the body. Good bacteria also ensure that toxins are excreted from the bowels instead of being absorbed into the bloodstream. **We now focus on four groups of compounds that can help to provide an ideal biological terrain in our bodies. They are digestive enzymes, probiotics, green foods and fiber.**

1. Digestive Enzymes

Our bodies contain more than 1,300 different types of enzymes. These enzymes act like construction workers building and maintaining our system. They are properly called molecule catalysts.

Enzymes come in several forms. They can be found in raw fruits and vegetables that are not very tasty to many of us. Cooking and food processing may improve the taste but they will destroy these important enzymes. Enzymes are destroyed when heated to 160°F. The body's ability to digest food, deliver up the nutrients and optimize bodily functions would be affected. Toxins will then begin to build up and accumulate in the body.

Digestive enzyme supplements are important when our body's natural supply is exhausted. Plant enzymes help in the digestion of food in the intestines and prevent a big bloated tummy after a big meal. Every day, our consumption of food totals approximately two pounds. For all these to be digested, we need a smooth passage of food through the gastrointestinal tract to avoid stasis of feces. This is where the digestive enzymes play an important role together with a high-fiber diet.

Digestive enzymes also help other vitamins and minerals. For example, the fat-soluble vitamins A, D, E, and K need fat for absorption. Fat has to be broken down by an enzyme known as lipase so that vitamins can be released. Consuming vitamin-rich food will be a waste of precious time and money if there are no proper enzymes to break down and release the vitamins into the body system.

In a cancer setting the use of digestive enzymes is critical. The relevant functions of these enzymes are:

- To attack the coating on tumor cells which disguise them from recognition by the immune system.
- To stimulate various components of the immune system such as natural killer cells, T-cells and tumor necrosis factor.
- To remove the "sticky" coating on cancer cells that allow them to attach themselves to other parts of the body. It prevents cancer spread.
- To penetrate cancer cells during their reproductive phase when they are not yet fully formed and to destroy them.
- To help ensure that large and potential allergy-triggering food particles do not enter the blood circulation through a leaky gut.
- To reduce the acidity of the internal terrain.

Therapeutic Dosage 1 tablet 3 to 4 times a day and then subsequently increasing to 5 tablets 4 times a day for advance cancers.

2. Probiotics

Probiotics are good bacteria as we previously stated. An excellent example of a good bacterium is *acidophilus. Acidophilus* stimulates activity in the thymus and spleen and prompt our bodies to produce natural antibodies. Some *acidophilus* strains also protect the body against cancers by helping to promote production of interferon, a hormone that protects against cancer.

Probiotics such as *acidophilus* also secrete mediators so that bad bacteria cannot grow. However, when the micro-organic forms take over, they will exclude the probiotics with their toxins. We can prevent this situation from arising through keeping our bowels healthy by populating it with probiotics. Probiotics that contain *lactobacillus acidophilus* and *bifidus* can aid in our body's detoxification program, for example.

In extensive and sophisticated studies conducted to assess the effectiveness of probiotics, the following have been concluded.

1. Probiotics can improve bowel transit time and the texture of the fecal matter.
2. It reduces lactose intolerance caused by a deficiency of lactase. The latter causes gas formation and bloating or stomach discomfort after milk consumption.
3. Probiotics can act as an anti-toxin with anti-carcinogenic and anti-tumor agents.
4. It helps to relieve dermatitis and other skin problems by improving gastrointestinal bacteria balance.

In addition to the above benefits, probiotics can also help to destroy toxins in other parts of the body besides the intestines. It is so strong that it can get rid of bad bacteria and fungi that produce their own toxins. Probiotics helps to minimize the risk of colon cancer, protects the whole body and improves general well-being.

Therapeutic Dosage Take probiotics such as *acidophilus* so as to repopulate our intestinal tract with good bacteria. At least 5 billion per serving, 2-4 times a day. *Acidophilus* supplements can be purchased in health and drugstores. When purchasing, select one that contain either *lactobacillus acidophilus, bifidobacterium bifidum, lactobacillus bulgaricus* or *streptococcus faecium.* All these are good bacteria. Do ensure that all purchases are fesh and well within the expiry date. These supplements are to be refrigerated. Any leftovers are to be thrown away after more than six months. Always consume those with the highest potency.

3. Green Foods

Green foods contain three algae and two cereal grasses. The algae are *chlorella*, *spirulina* and green blue algae. The grasses are wheat and barley grass. Green food is generally highly nutritious and *chlorella* is the most effective among the green food. They help to alkalinize the body and prevent cancer growth.

Chlorella is single-celled fresh water green algae that contain amino acids, enzymes, vitamins, minerals and carbohydrates. *Chlorella* is not only a self-contained whole food but also a complete protein source. It contains 18 of the 22 known amino acids including the eight essential amino acids.

Chlorella contains 50 to 60% proteins. Some other green foods also contain proteins. Their percentage of proteins is 73% in *spirulina*, 56% in blue green algae, 14% in barley grass and 18% in wheat grass. As such, *chlorella* contains a considerable proportion of proteins when compared with other green foods. It also has the highest concentration of chlorophyll in any plant. It has 5 to 10 times more than *spirulina*, wheat and barley grass. It is also higher in chlorophyll than the blue green algae. Chlorophyll is a powerful cleanser and detoxifier for the body.

Chlorella has been known to combat cancer. We will now look at some of its cancer-fighting properties.

- *Chlorella* stimulates interferon production. The latter is our body's natural immunity against cancer. *Chlorella*'s tough cell wall makes it a superior nutrient when comparing with other algae or grasses. Its cell wall can eliminate toxins, pesticides and heavy metals from the body.
- *Chlorella* growth factor is present in the nucleus. It enhances resistance to abdominal cancers by increasing the number of immune cells in the abdominal cavity. In studies where mice were fed *chlorella*, their life span was increased by over 30%.
- *Chlorella* increases T-Cells and B-Cells lymphocytes. White blood cell count is often improved.
- *Chlorella* helps to revitalize the body after chemotherapy. The patient is therefore less tired.

Notwithstanding its potency, *chlorella* does not enjoy celebrity status. Many people find it difficult to take *chlorella* on its own. In this case, they may wish to mix chlorella with vegetable juice or water and take it together with meals. However, do note that *chlorella* should not be mixed with fruit juice. Fruit juices are usually high in sugar content and lacks fiber.

Therapeutic Dosage To prevent cancer, 3 grams a day is recommended. Higher dosage at 10 to 30 grams a day is recommended for advance cancers. *Chlorella* can be taken at any time of the day. It can be taken all at once or in divided dosages throughout the day. So far, there is no known toxic dose. A word of caution, **since chlorella is a whole food, taking too much may not be good because of its detoxifying abilities leading to sudden toxic release.**

When chlorella is taken for the very first time, some people may experience cleansing reactions in the form of gas, cramping, constipation or diarrhea. Some may feel a "toxic release" sensation during the initial course. As such, very sensitive people may wish to begin with as little as 300 mg a day and gradually increasing the dose by 500 mg every 3 to 5 days.

4. Fiber

The average American's diet is very low in fiber. Many believe this is a key causative factor of colon cancer. We need to consume at least 25 to 30 grams daily for healthy bowel function. The consumption in Americans is reported to be only 5 to 15 grams a day. Clearly, this is not enough.

What's the solution then? Very simple. They can increase their fiber level by taking half a cup of bran, one cup of legume, two cups of vegetables, three fruits, whole grain bread and cereals on a daily basis. If they are fussy eaters, fiber supplementation together with digestive enzymes and drinking more water will also perform the same functions. These supplements are to be taken one hour before a meal so as not to interfere with the absorption of nutrients in the diet.

Fiber comes in two forms. They are soluble and insoluble fibers. Soluble fibers are found in fruits, oat bran, legumes, apple pectin and guar gum. *Psyllium* is an example that can be taken to control cholesterol.

Insoluble fibers are found in vegetables and whole grain products such as wheat bran. They assist in speeding food through the intestines. As such, the intestinal lining's exposure to food that may cause cancer is very much lessened. Cancer is prevented in this way.

Fiber can enhance good bacteria and reduce acidity in the digestive system, thus reducing the production of carcinogens. It is important to remember to drink plenty of water when taking soluble or insoluble fiber.

Therapeutic Dosage   15 to 35 grams of fiber a day to enhance digestive health and promote a smooth transit of food during digestion. Modified citrus pectin is a form of fiber that provides added protection to stop the spread of cancer cells. A compound called rhamnogalacturonan found in modified citrus pectin has a "bridging effect" that enhances the cytotoxic ability of T-lymphocytes. 15 grams a day is recommended.

CHAPTER **NINE**

UNLOAD YOUR TOXINS

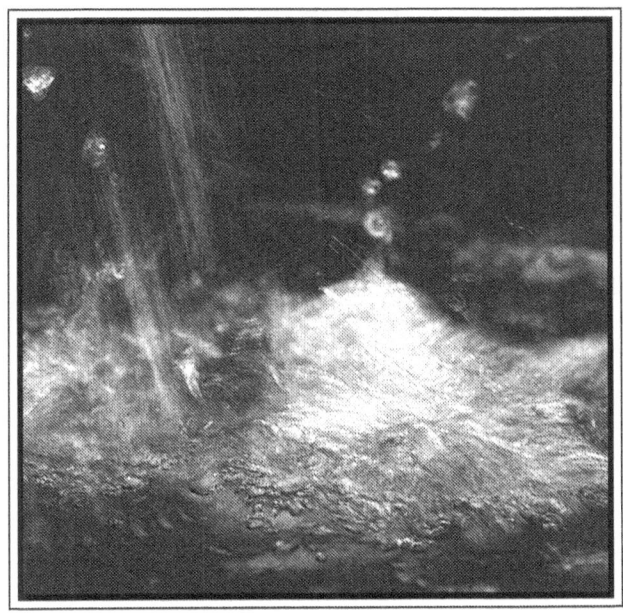

"The cleansing of toxins and waste products will
restore optimium function and vitality."

*Elson Haas, MD, director of the Marin Clinic
of Preventive Medicine and Health Education,
in* The Definitive Guide to Cancer

Exposure to an ever increasing array of toxic carcinogens in our air, food and water results in the production of cancer cells within the body. When our internal clearing system is unable to unload the toxin and the abnormal cells when they are few in number, cancer can result. The more toxins you have in your body, the faster will be the mutation of your healthy cells and the faster cancer will form.

One way of overcoming this problem is to identify ways of getting rid of these toxins from our bodies as early as possible.

Detoxification of the body means the cleansing of the bowels, kidneys, lungs, liver and blood. These are the vital organs that are involved in the elimination of chemicals and toxins from the body. Cancer stricken patients usually need intensive detoxification for several reasons. In the first place, their immune system succumbed to cancerous cells because of a highly toxic body at the onset. Then this toxicity is further compounded by the adverse effects of the toxins produced by the therapies used by conventional oncologists such as chemotherapy. Is there any wonder why cancer patients are often more sick than cured?

Most alternative cancer physicians believe that it is essential to flush all the toxins out of the body through major dietary changes and a multifaceted detoxification program that "cleans" the liver, kidney, lung, lymph, and skin.

Let us look at it more closely.

DEFINITION OF TOXINS

A toxin is defined as any compound that has a detrimental effect on cell function or structure.

Toxins can damage the body in an unseen and cumulative way. Toxic metabolites are formed when the body's internal detoxification system is overloaded. At this point, our bodies become more sensitive to other chemicals, some of which are normally not toxic. It is this accumulation of toxins over a period of time that can weaken our metabolic processes and result in a number of allergies and diseases.

Toxins are found in industrial chemicals, industrial wastes, pesticides, additives in our foods, heavy metals, anesthetics, drug residues, environmental hormones, and even secondary cigarette smoke. There are altogether two million synthetic substances and 25,000 new toxins are added each year. This means that the world is becoming more and more toxic at a really alarming rate!

When we are exposed to toxins for a long time, our body cells are affected. The toxins are carcinogenic as they alter human DNA. Even the World Health Organization has identified the problem and it blames environmental toxic chemicals for causing the cancer and much havoc in our surroundings.

TYPES OF TOXINS

The types of toxins are classified into the following categories:

1. Toxic metals
2. Liver toxins
3. Microbial toxins
4. Protein by-product toxins

1. Toxic Metals

Toxic metals including lead, mercury, cadmium, arsenic, nickel and aluminum are most likely to accumulate in the brain, kidneys and immune system.

About 25% of the US population suffers from heavy metal poisoning. Believe it or not, every year, over 600,000 tons of lead are released into the environment from industrial processes and leaded gasoline. The toxins are either inhaled or ingested after being absorbed into food crops, fresh water and soil.

Other sources of toxic metals are from pesticide sprays, cadmium batteries, cigarette smoke, mercury in dental fillings, contaminated fish, aluminum from antacids, cookware and soda cans.

The level of toxins in our bodies can be assessed by a blood analysis of the actual toxin level of each metal within the red blood cell. Many toxic metals have a tendency to accumulate inside the cell, where most of the damage is done. The commonly used measures of extracellular serum toxic metal levels are therefore seldom accurate.

Toxic metals cause Alzheimer's disease, Parkinson's disease and severe neurological disorders. If you are poisoned by heavy metals, chances are that you will suffer from headaches, fatigue, muscle pain, indigestion, constipation, anemia, and tremors. Mild toxicity symptoms include impaired memory and distorted thinking. You can even die of severe metal poisoning.

We can rectify the above problem by using chelation therapy to bind toxic metals, or taking high potency vitamin and mineral supplements including vitamins C and B complex and sulfur-containing amino acids. We must also increase our intake of high sulfur-content food such as garlic, onion, eggs, guar gum, oat bran, pectin and *psyllium* seeds.

2. Liver Toxins

Our liver is the major detoxification center of the body. It filters unwanted substances and wastes from the blood and gets rid of toxins such as alcohol, solvents, formaldehyde, pesticides, herbicides and food additives. The liver can also reduce toxins to compounds that can be safely removed via the kidney as urine, the skin as sweat, the lungs as expelled air and the bowels as feces. As the liver plays such an important function, we must ensure it remains healthy.

The symptoms of heavy metal poisoning in the liver include psychological and neurological conditions manifested as depression, headache, confusion, mental illness, abnormal nerve reflexes and tremor in the hands.

To detoxify the liver, we can take compounds such as milk thistle extract, choline, methionine and antioxidants.

3. Microbial Toxins

As stated earlier, there are good and bad microbes in our system. The bad ones secrete harmful substances. So how do you prevent your intestines from absorbing toxins that will lead to disastrous effects in your body?

Some of these toxins include endotoxins and exotoxins from bacteria, toxic amines, toxic derivatives from bile and many other carcinogens. When the intestines absorb these toxins, you might develop conditions such as Crohn's disease, ulcerative colitis, liver disease, psoriasis, lupus, pancreatitis, allergies, asthma and immune disorders.

When antibodies are formed against antigens, they can "cross-react" with the body's cells. This causes auto-immune diseases such as rheumatoid arthritis, myasthenia gravis, diabetes and auto-immune thyroiditis.

Take more soluble fibers such as those found in fruits, guar gum, pectin and oat bran to solve this problem. Fiber can help to eliminate toxins from the intestines and promote their excretion.

4. Protein By-product Toxins

Our kidney is the other key player responsible for the elimination of toxic waste products such as ammonia and urea from protein breakdown.

Detoxification of the body involves **cleansing the kidney with plenty of water.** Water is often regarded as the fountain of life. So, take more of it if you wish to live longer. Have at least 8 to 10 glasses of filtered water a day.

Cut down on meats, dairy products and other proteins and this will prevent overloading the body with urea which is a waste product that should be gotten rid of.

DO WE NEED DETOXIFICATION?

As long as we are on this earth, we will not be able to find a safe haven free from toxins and pollutants. The air that we breathe is polluted, the water that we drink is full of chlorine and the clothing we wear is made from artificial fabrics and chemicals. In every household, the lotions, cleaning detergents, soaps and shampoos all contain toxic chemicals. Many of us are not even aware that these products contain harmful toxins. When we absorb these chemicals, be it directly or indirectly, we can never eliminate them fully unless we undergo a detoxification process. Everybody needs some form of detoxification. It is the only way to survive this polluted and toxic environment.

Our bodies are created to be self-cleansing and self-healing. The internal detoxification process is an automatic daily routine via the major detoxification organs. Today, our toxic environment is overloading our detoxification system. So health-conscious individuals are choosing detoxification processes to maintain their bodies.

Detoxification is a key component in any comprehensive cancer program. In a cancer setting, an intensive detoxification program usually requires three to four weeks of intravenous solutions, diet adjustments and enemas. It is very effective and many spontaneous cancers have been controlled by detoxification alone.

Benefits of Detoxification

These are some of the benefits of detoxifications:

1. The digestive tract is cleansed of accumulated waste and fermenting bacteria.
2. Liver, kidney and blood purification can take place. The natural purification process would have been compromised by the toxins.
3. Mental clarity is enhanced as chemicals and food additives are eliminated.
4. The dependency on sugar, caffeine, nicotine, alcohol and drugs is reduced.
5. The immune system is stimulated.

PRINCIPLES OF A DETOXIFICATION PROGRAM

There are three basic principles of a detoxification program.

1. Cleansing
2. Rebuilding
3. Maintenance

1. Cleansing

There are many forms of cleansing. Cleansing of the body system can be achieved internally through fasting and externally through skin cleansing. The other ways are vegetable juicing, colon cleansing, kidney cleansing, lung cleansing and toxic metal cleansing. These will be examined in detail below. In some cases, enemas are used but they are normally reserved for cases where intense cleansing is required.

A. Complete Fasting

Complete fasting **is not recommended** for the cancer patient unless the patient is in remission and in good health. The reason is simple, the cancer patient needs all the good nutrition he or she can get. While a complete fast is a wonderful way to detoxify, we do not want the detoxification process to further weaken the body that is already suffering from the toxic drugs and chemotherapeutic agents onboard.

B. Vegetable Juicing

The vegetable juice fast is an effective form of cleansing. Vegetable juices are excellent sources of vitamins, minerals and enzymes.

This is also an **excellent form of detoxification for cancer patients.** They should benefit from a high dose of vegetable juices for their nutrition and antioxidant effects. However, the cancer patient should exercise caution when undergoing this form of fasting. They should be under supervision by their doctor.

Fruit and vegetable juices are a world apart. Although vegetable juices are one of the most unappreciated choices, they actually contain good sources of antioxidants and enzymes needed for toxin cleansing and excretion. They are easy to digest, nutritious and help to get rid of indigestion.

Certain vegetables should be taken in small amounts due to their high sugar content. Carrots and beetroots, for example fall into this category. They increase the blood sugar level considerably. As vegetable juices do not taste as nice as fruit juices, small amounts like one or two ounces each time, may be drunk initially. This amount should be gradually increased to 12 ounces without causing any nausea or belching.

Whole vegetables should also be taken together with the vegetable juices or after the drink. This is important because the chewing motion of eating vegetables will stimulate gastric juice secretion and promote digestion.

The best part of the juice is the pulp. It provides bulk and fiber to our diet and aids bowel movements. The only drawback is that it does not taste too good. We can try mixing a small amount into the juice first and then gradually increasing it when we are used to the taste. Not many people can consume all the pulp with the juice. It is quite thick and will probably look like a bowl of porridge instead of a glass of juice.

Vegetable juice should be **consumed immediately** as its nutrients are very perishable. As far as possible do not keep it for more than 24 hours. For storing vegetable juice, use a glass jar with an airtight lid. Fill the juice to the brim to minimize air space because oxygen in the air pocket will oxidize and damage the juice. Thereafter, wrap the jar with aluminum foil to block out all light and then store it in the refrigerator. Remove the juice from the refrigerator 30 minutes before drinking so as to allow it to be consumed at room temperature.

Beginners may wish to start with juicing celery, fennel (anise) and cucumbers. This combination tastes rather good. Later, they can be motivated to include other vegetables and herbs such as spinach, cabbage, bok choy, endive, lettuce, parsley and cilantro. The advance juice drinker should consider collard green, dandelion green and mustard green as these vegetables are very beneficial. They taste bitter but they are good for you.

Sometimes, a little carrot and beetroot can be added to these bitter juices. However, the amount should be minimal as they are higher in sugar content when compared with their green leafy counterparts. Try adding a little lemon juice as it is a strong blood alkalizer. When alkalinity is raised in the blood stream, calcium ion is reduced. This is good because calcium ion enhances tumor growth.

Cancer patients should minimize their intake of fruit juices and take more vegetable juices. Fruit juices contain too much sugar and this will increase the patient's blood sugar and insulin levels. Remember cancer cells thrive in a sugar environment. If fruit juice has to be taken, then it should be diluted with water.

C. Skin Cleanse

Sweating helps to release toxins from our bodies. As our skin is one of the most effective excretion organs, a detoxification program emphasizing skin cleansing is essential. Our sweat glands team up with our kidneys to effectively perform the detoxification.

Good skin care is important. Many of us do not know that "skin care" products such as soaps and shampoos contain deadly synthetic chemicals. Unknowingly, we are being poisoned as we bathe, as more toxins are absorbed into our bodies. We are not aware of the dangers that we can't see so long as our liver is able to metabolize these toxins. To avoid being poisoned, consider switching to natural soaps and shampoos. These contain no toxins and chemicals.

Exercise, sauna, skin brushing and detoxification baths can remove such toxins. Let us take a closer look at these methods.

i. Skin Brushing

Keep brushing your skin to remove the outer dead skin layers and keep your pores open! After bathing, we can try using the towel to give our skin a good scrub until it is slightly red. Do note that these towels will have to be changed regularly as they may contain toxins from the scrubbing.

ii. Sauna Bath

These very popular methods are excellent ways of removing toxins from the skin. They also rejuvenate our health and energy level. It is good to go into the sauna after dry skin brushing as the intense heat encourages excessive sweating and removes toxins in the process. Regular sauna treatment is an excellent detoxification tool, especially for the cancer patient for the simple reason that cancer cells do not handle heat as well as regular cells. Do not stay inside the sauna too long as it can cause excessive dehydration.

iii. Detoxification Baths

These are baths using natural soaps and oils. They are very effective in removing toxins from our bodies. It is important to use only natural soaps and oils to do this.

Try this method. Use 1/2 cup of baking soda, 1/2 cup of epsom salt or 1/2 cup of sea salt. Add these into the bath water. Then, soak for 15 to 20 minutes. Scrub the skin gently with natural soap. The water will turn murky and dirty within minutes as the heavy metals are excreted from the skin. Immersing in a Jacuzzi bath with added hydrogen peroxide or ozone is also invigorating and makes a good start for the day.

It is important to purchase a filter for our shower as more toxins are absorbed during bathing than from drinking tap water. We should also avoid swimming in a chlorinated swimming pool. Go to the beach and swim in the ocean instead.

D. Colon Cleanse

This method is one of the oldest forms of detoxification as it has been used for 4,000 years. Colon cleansing can heal, rebuild and restore the colon's size and functions.

Colon cleansing works by flushing the colon with a warm water solution. It protects our bodies by removing toxins that may lead to cancer, colitis, digestive disorders, fatigue and obesity.

There are two stages in this therapy. The first stage involves a thorough cleaning of the colon. Water is pumped in gently and allowed to flow in and out at steady intervals. The water moves through the entire length of the colon and also around the cecum. During this process, the walls of the colon are washed. Any old encrustations and fecal material are loosened, dislodged and flushed away. These toxic waste materials may have been attached to the walls for several years. They contain millions of bacteria that can lead to cancer and many other serious diseases.

Colon cleansing helps to treat diseases such as severe skin disorders, breathing difficulties, depression, chronic fatigue, nervousness, severe constipation and arthritis. Together with a change in diet and other forms of treatment, the patient will feel much better.

After colon cleansing, the next stage is healing, rebuilding and restoration of a healthy colon. During the healing phase, a special liquid is poured into the bowel to cool inflamed areas and strengthen weak sections of the colon wall. Some of the agents used during this healing stage are flaxseed tea, white oak bark and slippery elm bark. These herbs soothe and lubricate the colon. In some cases, herbal teas are also taken during colon cleansing. But one thing we must not forget in this entire process is to drink plenty of water.

Probiotics are often added to ensure that beneficial flora remains in positive balance through out the gastrointestinal tract.

The mention of enema makes many people feel disgusted and uncomfortable. This notion must be dispelled. In actual fact, it is a very quick and effective way of loosening impacted feces and washing them away. It also removes the unpleasant symptoms of detoxification.

Alternatively, we can consider a colon cleansing diet. Begin with a diet of 50% raw food along with a teaspoonful of linseed or two level teaspoonfuls of metamucil. The linseed can also be chewed orally to release the nutrients. Remember to drink plenty of water before breakfast and throughout the day. The water intake should be at least two quarts per day during the cleansing period.

E. Lung and Lymphatic Cleanse

Cancer cells can't survive in a high-oxygen environment. Using this fact, we can prevent cancer by doing aerobics exercises and other forms of exercises to help cleanse the lungs and enrich the body's oxygen intake. When we exercise, the bad air that is trapped in our lungs is forced out in exchange for fresh air. The bad air is trapped in the small alveoli in the lungs and can only be expelled during exercise.

Exercise at least 30 minutes a day if it can be tolerated. This can be broken down into 5- to 10-minute sessions. If you are weak, simply go for a stroll in the park or jog slowly to keep the optimal oxygen circulation, promote detoxification of the lungs and promote lymphatic drainage.

Try to exercise in less polluted areas like the park or gardens that are away from industrial buildings and heavily utilized roads. Our regime should include breathing exercises to increase the action of lymphatic cleansing. We can do this by synchronizing our breathing with our body movements during exercise. For example, when we are walking or jumping on the trampoline, we can inhale four times and exhale four times rhythmically. Breathe in through our nose and exhale through our nose or mouth. A 10-minute deep breathing exercise can be helpful.

The lymphatic system drains away toxins and cancer cells. **Lymphatic massage or lymphatic drainage machines can enhance it.**

F. Kidney and Blood Cleanse

Drink your way to good health. **Drink a quart of pure filtered water for every 50 pounds of your body weight.** But regardless, everyone, young and old, should drink at least 10 to15 glasses of filtered or bottled water daily.

Drinking the right type of water is important. Distilled water comes from a process in which water is boiled, evaporated and the vapor condensed. It has no dissolved minerals and can absorb toxic substances from the body and eliminate them. Distilled water is taken during detoxification for a brief period to help the body eliminate unwanted minerals. Once this is accomplished, the consumption of distilled water should be stopped.

Too much distilled water over a long time can be dangerous as the rapid loss of sodium, potassium, chloride and trace minerals cause multiple mineral deficiencies. Furthermore, it can also over-acidify the body. When exposed to air, distilled water absorbs carbon dioxide in the air and becomes acidic with a pH as low as 5.8. (pH of ordinary water is around 7.)

The best drinking water should be slightly alkaline and contain minerals such as calcium and magnesium. Water that has been filtered through a carbon block or reverse osmosis tends to be neutral. This is ideal for long-term consumption.

We have to ensure that our filters can remove pollutants and parasites such as *cryptosporidium*. Bottled water may be the next best option if we do not have a filter in our home. However, it has been noted that about 25 to 30% of bottled water sold in the United States comes from tap water that may not be treated.

What Kind of Water Should You Drink?

- The Best: Pure Filtered Water
- Second Best: Bottled Water
- Use Sparingly: Distilled Water
- Avoid: Tap Water

Willard's Water

This is a form of mineral water that contains magnesium sulfate, sulfated castor oil, sodium silicate and powdered lignite. A patented catalyst usually alters the water.

Willard's water is prepared by mixing an ounce of the Willard's water concentrate with a gallon of filtered water. It acts as an antioxidant, an alkalizer and a detoxifier. The pH level of Willard's water is 12.5. Water mixed this way with Willard's water has a pH of 10.4. Some forms of Willard's water contain lignite coal, which is a natural detoxifier.

Some studies have reported that after drinking this water, toxic metal was found in the test subject's urine. This means that Willard's water may assist in the detoxification of heavy metals. How much can a cancer patient drink in a day? There is no reported limit on the amount of Willard's water one can consume.

G. Toxic Metal Cleanse

Toxic metals prevent normal enzymatic processes. As a result, the body cannot function properly and repair itself. This leads to premature aging and the early development of disease including cancer. It is therefore important to detoxify our bodies to get rid of such toxic metals.

We can do this through chelation therapy. In this therapy, toxic metals are removed to allow the body to function at an optimum level. During the chelation process, a synthetic amino acid called EDTA is given to the patient by intravenous bolus or drip. Different clinicians uses different techniques. One session generally runs from 2 to 3 hours when 1.5 to 3 grams of sodium EDTA is used. Some clinicians use calcium-EDTA instead and is able to deliver the necessary 1.5- 3 grams chelating agent in a matter of minutes with an IV push. Once the EDTA enters the blood stream, it binds to heavy metals such as cadmium, lead, arsenic, and to a lesser degree, mercury. Toxic metals are damaging to the endothelial wall of the blood vessel. Damaged endothelial wall is unable to secrete a vasodilator called nitrous oxide. Without nitrous oxide, the vessel constricts, leading to high blood pressure, increased shearing force of blood flow, and a cascade of events known as inflammatory response as the body tries to overcome this abnormal condition. In this inflammatory response, the body mobilizes white blood cells and macrophages (also called foam cells). Foam cells deposit in the endothelium and attract oxidized LDL cholesterol. Such oxidized LDL cholesterol in turn attracts other cholesterol of the same, eventually leading to the formation of soft artherosclerotic plaques and cardio-vascular accidents.

As toxic metals are removed, the endothelium insult is reduced, and blood vessel is able to secrete the vasodilator nitrous oxide. The vessel is relaxed, the lumen size enlarges, and blood flow is increased. As a result blood pressure is normalized and the risk of cardiovascular accident reduces.

2. Rebuilding

A rebuilding detoxification diet enhances the body's immune system. This process takes place after cleansing. The body can only be rebuilt with the proper raw materials. One way is to adopt a healthy diet and adhere strictly to it.

A rebuilding detoxification diet is essentially vegetarian consisting of whole fruits, green leafy vegetables, legumes and seeds. A limited amount of fish intake may be permitted. Organic eggs can be eaten but in reasonable quantities. During the detoxification program, food groups are rotated every four days. This allows maximum elimination from the body before another quantity of the same food group is ingested.

3. Maintenance

After detoxification, we should keep our bodies clean and toxin free. A healthy lifestyle must include exercise, diet, supplementation, stress reduction, hormonal enhancement and a regular intake of cleansing herbal teas.

Cleansing Herbal Teas

Found in the form of teas, powders or extracts, non-caffeinated herbal tea such as senna leaf, peppermint leaf, steria leaf, buckthorn bark, damiana leaf, red peel, chamomile flower and uva ursi leaf. Cleansing tea is gentle and mild and can be consumed regularly to keep the body cleansed. Herbal teas do not contain caffeine. Herbal cleansing tea in powder form also comes in a capsule for easier swallowing. They are best taken with meals and digestive enzymes. However, do note that herbal extracts with alcohol content should be avoided.

Here is a good example of a simple herbal cleansing program that can be used in conjunction with a detoxification diet.

1. Have a good night's sleep and rise early.
2. Drink a glass of lemon water or plain water with a teaspoon of apple cider vinegar and a teaspoon of blackstrap molasses.

3. In the later part of the morning, drink a glass of plain water with added *psyllium* husk powder, followed by another glass of water.
4. Take two to three multi-digestive enzymes and liver herbs during the three main meals.
5. Drink plenty of herbal cleansing teas in between meals to support the liver.

THE GERSON THERAPY OF DETOXIFICATION

This therapy was mentioned in the introductory section of this book. The treatment is designed for cancer patients.

This therapy was founded by the distinguished Dr Max Gerson. Born and bred in Germany in 1881, Dr Gerson began his quest for a drug to cure migraine. You see, he was suffering from very bad migraine. After searching and experimenting for a period of time, he invented the Gerson Therapy of Detoxification. Later, he discovered that this treatment not only cured his severe migraines, it also cured his skin tuberculosis. He felt very excited about this fluke discovery and decided to use this special detoxification diet to treat many tuberculosis patients. He managed to cure many patients and became very successful.

A few years later, Dr Gerson used the same therapy on Dr Albert Schweitzer's wife who was afflicted with incurable lung tuberculosis. Her condition was diagnosed as very serious and there was nothing much doctors could do to save her. After Dr Gerson placed her on his program, she began to show signs of recovery. There was hope. She miraculously recovered and continued to live on till old age. Later, Dr Gerson and Dr Schweitzer continued to do more research on this therapy and discovered that this dietary therapy was also successful in treating heart disease, kidney failure and cancer.

The Gerson Therapy is a program of natural detoxification involving:

1. Detoxification of the whole body.
2. Fortifying the body with potassium. Cancer patients have too much sodium compared to potassium in their bodies. Sodium acts as a poison in the body because it is an enzyme inhibitor. Potassium is an enzyme activator.
3. Taking oxidizing enzymes in the form of green leaf juice and calf liver juice until the body can produce them on their own.

The Gerson Therapy restores the normal condition of the oxidizing system in the body so that cancer cells cannot function. The objective in this therapy is to boost the body's immune system and cure cancer, arthritis, heart disease, allergies, and many other old-age diseases.

The patients take plenty of nutrients from the juice of 13 organically grown vegetables daily. They are taken at intensive intervals of every two hours around the clock during the therapy. This intake provides the body with a mega dose of enzymes, minerals and nutrients and helps to break down the bad cells in the body. At the same time, coffee enemas also used in this therapy will aid in removing the lifelong buildup of toxins from the liver. The Gerson Therapy has celebrated high success over the past 60 years. Many people were miraculously cured after going through this program. It also boasts of its success in treating melanoma, lymphoma, ovarian cancer, colorectal cancer, lupus and arthritis.

CHAPTER TEN

ANTI-CANCER DIET

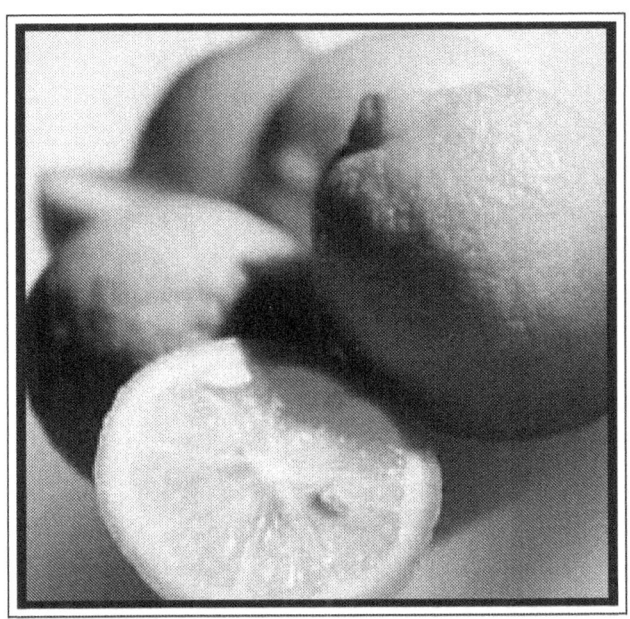

There is an abundance of scientific evidence showing that
a clinically guided nutrition program for the cancer patient…can
improve quality of life by 12 to 21 fold…
and a greater likelihood of complete remission."

Patrick Quillin, PhD, in Beating Cancer with Nutrition.

W e live in a world of over-calorie and under-nutrition. Sadly the statistics show that 74% of Americans are below daily RDA requirements for magnesium, 55% for iron, 68% calcium, 40% vitamin C, 33% vitamin B12, 80% B6, 33% B3, 35% B2, 45% B1, and 50% vitamin A.

According to Patrick Quillin, PhD, author of *Beating Cancer with Nutrition,*

> *25 to 50% of hospital patients suffer from protein calorie malnutrition. Pure malnutrition (cachexia) is responsible for at least 22% and up to 67% of all cancer deaths. Up to 80% of all cancer patients have reduced levels of serum albumin, which is a leading indicator of protein and calorie malnutrition. At least 20% of Americans are clinically malnourished, with 70% being sub-clinically malnourished, and the remaining 'chosen few' 10% in good optimal health.*

For decades, physicians learned and people are told that daily diet provides all the necessary nutrients one will need for a healthy life. This is no longer true today. We now know that **food alone simply cannot supply all the nutrients that our body needs for optimum health,** let alone the dosage and level used as a modality for the reversal of disease such as cancer. Moreover, today's food is devoid of many minerals and vitamins compared to those a few decades ago. This is probably because of the changing environment and pollution.

Today, nutritional science is used by many forward-looking physicians. Nutritional cancer therapy is now a mainstream medical movement in the United States and Canada. It is supported by doctors from the Harvard School of Medicine, National Cancer Institute and National Institutes of Health. Some high-profiled doctors such as Dr Charles Simone, the oncologist to President Reagan, and Dr Abram Hoffer, a chief collaborator with Linus Pauling, have also endorsed this treatment. If only doctors had embraced this concept much earlier, more lives could have been saved.

While conventional therapies weaken the body over time, alternative non-toxic nutritional therapies build up the body's anti-cancer defense. Many miraculous recoveries from cancer have been reported from this form of treatment. A study reported that **88% of spontaneous remission involves significant dietary change and the intake of nutritional supplementation and herbs.**

Is there any surprise that poor nutrition is a major causative factor in cancer? Nutrition is the foundation of health and a cornerstone in cancer therapy. In fact, malnutrition alone kills 40% of cancer patients as we have mentioned earlier. Nutrition therefore plays the critical part of a complete non-toxic natural therapeutic program for treating cancer.

BENEFITS OF A GOOD DIET

You take in an average of over 20 tons of food in a lifetime. You are literally what you eat.

There is no doubt that a good diet increases the cancer patient's lifespan. An optimum level of nutrients fights cancer in many different ways.

1. Free radical regulators. A high-sugar diet leads to vitamin C depletion as the body uses endogenous vitamin C as an antioxidant to overcome the free radical damage of sugar. Excessive free radical damage therefore results in vitamin C deficiency.

2. Nutrients are able to change cell membrane dynamics where most hormone receptors are located. The fat in the diet dictates the composition of this lipid bilayer. Omega-3 fatty acid from fish

oil and GLA from borage oil enhance cell membranes to increase receptor sensitivity to insulin and prevent insulin resistance. Insulin resistance afflicts over 60 million Americans and has been linked to a variety of cancers.

CHARACTERISTICS OF AN ANTI-CANCER DIET

1. Low in Sugar

Cancer lives well in a sugar environment. They use sugar as a form of fuel instead of oxygen. As such, a diet rich in sugar will promote cancer cell growth and reduce our immune function. Studies have shown that animals that are fed a low-sugar diet have a 95% chance of survival after injection of mammary tumor into their bodies. Animals that were a fed high-sugar diet only had a survival rate of 33%. Clearly, sugar is a silent killer.

Over the past century, the consumption of refined sugar has increased from 60 to 180 pounds a year per person. Today's generation seems to be taking in more sugar in various forms. Scientist Dr Warburg said that cancers exhibit an increase in anaerobic glycolysis. This is a process whereby glucose is used as a fuel by cancer cells with lactic acid as by-product. Cancer cells contain three times as much insulin as normal cells. A sugarless diet is therefore a key component of any cancer diet. With no sugar, the cancer cells cannot thrive. It is important to starve the cancer cell by taking less sugar and more whole foods, fresh vegetables and vegetable juice. We should also refrain from animal products or by-products as these products are high in saturated fats and promote cancer. Sugar can also be found in potato, white bread, pastas and corn.

We will now look at a few examples. A study using a mouse model of human breast cancer shows that tumors are sensitive to glucose. In the study, 68 mice were injected with an aggressive strain of breast cancer and then fed diets to induce high, normal or low blood sugar. The results showed that the lower the sugar level, the higher the survival rate.

Another study of four years was conducted at the National Institute of Public Health and Environmental Protection in the Netherlands. A group comprising 111 biliary tract cancer patients was compared with a control group of 480 people. The study showed similar results that proved that a higher cancer risk was related to a high intake of sugar.

In another epidemiological study in 21 developed countries, it was reported that sugar intake is a strong risk factor that contributes to higher breast cancer rates.

All cancer patients must reduce their sugar intake. It will surely slow down the effects and invasiveness of cancer. We are not implying that sugar should be avoided totally. A certain amount of sugar is needed for basic function. Instead, we should ensure that our blood glucose is within a narrow range to help starve the cancer cells and boost immune functions.

Glycemic Index

Glycemic index is a measure of how fast a food increases the blood sugar. Controlling blood sugar is one of the key pillars in a successful anti-cancer diet. High blood sugar and high triglyceride are both direct reflections of high sugar. Knowing what low sugar food to take is important. Concentrate on food with an index of under 70 and preferably under 60. Good choices include basmati rice, oats, millet and bailey.

Here is a table of common foods and their glycemic index. To reduce blood sugar handling stress, concentrate on foods with an index at or below 75. This will help create a more even flow of glucose into the blood. If you are taking high-glycemic index food like white bread, always try to mix it up low-glycemic index food to average out their indexes.

GLYCEMIC INDEX

Grain and Cereal Products		Vegetables	
White Rice, Short Grain	83	Baked Potato	85
White Bread	70	White Potato	82
Whole Wheat Bread	70	Sweet Potato	61
Brown Rice, Long Grain	50	New Potato	58
Rye Bread	50	Corn	54
White Spaghetti	40	Carrot	47
Wheat Spaghetti	37	Yam	37

Breakfast Cereals		Legumes	
Cornflakes	92	Baked Beans	60
Puffed Rice	82	Soybeans	48
Shredded Wheat	80	Peas (dried)	32
Grape Nut	78	Butter Beans	31
Oatmeal (regular)	49	Lentils	29
All Bran	38	Kidney Beans	28
		Chickpeas	28

Fruits		Dairy Products	
Watermelon	72	Ice cream	62
Raisin	64	Yogurt	36
Banana	52	Whole Milk	34
Mango	51	Skim Milk	32
Orange Juice	46		
Grape	45		
Orange	40	**Sweeteners**	
Apple	39	Maltose	152
Plum	39	Glucose	100
Pear	38	Honey	87
Peach	38	Sucrose	86
Grapefruit	26	Fructose	20

Adapted from D.J.A. Jenkins et. al., American Journal of Clinical Nutrition, Volume 34, 1981

2. High in Antioxidants

Most green leafy vegetables are high in antioxidants. The more colorful the vegetable, the higher the level. Broccoli, spinach, bok choy are particularly good choices. Be careful to refrain from eating vegetables that grow underground, such as potato or carrots as these are high in starch and sugar. These are vegetables but behave like a grain and turn quickly into sugar when inside our body.

Dietary antioxidant in high doses have been shown to enhance chemotherapy and radiotherapy agents if given in series on a daily basis during the course of chemo- and radiotherapy. Some nutrients, too, augment the effect of chemotherapeutic agents. Studies have shown that high doses of vitamin C, beta-carotene, and vitamin E succinate, can cause a 50% reduction in melanoma cell growth, while there is no effect on normal cells. In selected cases such as colon cancer, vitamin E has been shown to be more effective than 5FU in reducing cancer cell based on laboratory animal models. Antioxidants also increase the effect of hyperthermia without affecting the normal cell.

3. Promoters of an Alkaline Environment

We have said that cancer cells thrive in an acidic environment.

The three primary generators of acid in a cancer patient are:

1. **The metabolism and/or incomplete breakdown (oxidation) of foodstuffs or metabolic "wastes"** as a by-product of cellular activity. During normal cellular respiration and energy production, acids are produced as part of these "waste" products. These acids must be "balanced", neutralized, or removed by the body's buffering and detoxification systems through the kidneys, lungs, liver and blood. In the case of a cancer patient, this is even more prevalent as cancer cells take in sugar as fuel and release lactic acid as waste.

2. **The consumption of acid present in food, air, and drinking water.** Nitrogen emissions from automobiles and industrial plants, food dyes, sprays, waxes, preservatives, additives, artificial sweeteners, fertilizers, water pollutants, and even the chlorides and fluorides in tap water are just some of the highly acidic chemicals ingested by millions everyday.

Foods are generally broken down and converted into either acidic or alkaline substrates with digestion. **A person with an acidic metabolic condition should step up his consumption of alkali-forming foods daily, with 60-70% alkali-forming foods, and 30-40% acid-forming food by volume.**

Do not mistakenly eat all alkali-forming food alone, as some acid formation is necessary to generate metabolic activity and maintain homeostasis. Too alkaline a body can predispose the body to certain types of infection.

Here are some of the common acid and alkali forming foods. These categories are based on the body's reaction to a moderate amount of each. Excess amounts may produce the opposite effect.

Acid-Producing Foods

most grains	pasta	eggs	most chemicals and drugs
most beans	fish	dairy	sugar, saccharin,
meat	fowl	red meat	tobacco, soft drinks
tempeh	nuts	vinegar	most alcoholic beverages
			coffee, tea, beer

Alkali-Producing Foods

miso	sea salt	yeast	fruits (except cranberry, blueberry,
millet	soy sauce	seaweed	prune, plum)
seeds	green soy bean		soda water
sprouts	lima bean		
tofu	green pea		

Alkali-Producing Vegetables

- green leafy vegetables (watercress, spinach, kale, etc.)

- below the ground type "root" vegetables (carrot, turnip, onion etc.)

- other above ground vegetables (broccoli, cauliflower, squash, cucumber etc.)

4. Promoters of the Immune System

Good nutrition leads to a strong immune system. The foods that promote such a system include garlic, onions, grapes, tomatoes, and broccoli. There is little doubt that a high sugar environment retards the immune system.

WHERE IS THE EVIDENCE?

The evidence is in the following case studies.

1. In 1995, a study with a sampling group of 48,000 men reported that those who ate 10 servings of tomato-rich foods every week reduced their risk of prostate cancer by 50%.

2. It is common for men to have pre-cancerous prostate lesions. In the United States, the rate of advance prostate cancer is six times more then the rate in Japan. The average American's diet contains 40% of fat whilst the Japanese's diet only has 20% of it. This clearly shows that fat consumption increases the risk of prostate cancer.

3. Animal studies have shown that tumor cells are less aggressive in animals on a low-fat diet than in those fed a higher-fat diet.

4. A study was conducted with a large sampling group of 83,000 women. Their ages were between 33 to 60 years. It was reported that consumption of fruits and vegetables high in specific carotenoids and vitamins had a significant reduction in premenopausal breast cancer risk. This was especially so when there was a family history of breast cancer.

WHAT FOOD TO EAT?

Include plenty of green leafy vegetables, water, legume, whole grain, seeds and essential fats in your everyday healthy diet. These foods are often quite under-rated.

How then should we go about choosing a well-balanced diet? Here's a guide. A normal meal should contain 25% lean or plant protein, 35% cooked plant food such as beans, whole grain bread or whole grain tortilla and 40% raw vegetables such as broccoli, spinach, tomato and raw fruits.

When choosing what food to consume, we should take note of the following factors.

- Raw food and moderately cooked food is more beneficial. Select the ones that are of low-glycemic index. For example, we should take pureed carrots instead of carrot juice.
- Take fresh low-glycemic organic fruits Some examples are apples, apricots, currants, nectarines, peaches, plums and pineapples.
- Sprouted and cooked cereal grains are good. These include oats, basmati rice, millet, rye, barley and buckwheat.
- Eat vegetable protein instead of animal protein. Vegetable proteins include legumes such as lentils, chickpeas, kidney beans, lima beans and green peas, nuts and seeds.
- **Refrain from cooking with unsaturated oils and margarine totally.** Instead, take butter and olive oil.
- Coffee intake should be restricted. Switch to decaffeinated coffee and a maximum of one cup a day. The best is to refrain from coffee totally.
- Heavy meals are to be avoided at night.
- Do not combine fruits with concentrated proteins in the same meal that may produce gas and discomfort.

- **Drink two pints of freshly made vegetable juice per day.** This should include combinations of endive, lettuce, cabbage, celery, parsley and spinach. Carrot or beetroot are high in sugar content. Small amounts are acceptable. Include some of the pulps in the juice.
- **Citrus fruits are not recommended for every patient.** Sometimes, fresh oranges or grapefruit can be taken in between meals. Citrus fruit juice and vegetable juice should not be consumed within one hour of a meal. The exception is lemon and lime. Add 1/3 to 1/2 cup of lemon juice to each meal. The juice should be poured over the meal or consumed directly in a cup of water to aid digestion. Lemon juice is a rich source of citric acid and potassium. When combined with potassium citrate, it is one of the strongest blood alkalizers.
- All fruits, vegetables, fish and meat should be washed in a diluted 3% solution of hydrogen peroxide or given a 20-minute wash in an ozonated water bath help to remove bacteria on the food.
- **Flaxseed or cold-pressed and unrefined flaxseed oil** is an excellent source of dietary fat. More than 60% of flaxseed oil is alpha-linolenic acid. This acid is a form of omega-3 fatty acid that our bodies require for immunity boosting. Flaxseed should not be heated as heating will cause free radicals to be formed. It should be mixed directly with sulfur-rich foods such as legumes. The recommended dose is 1 to 2 tablespoon daily.
- **Animal protein especially commercially grown poultry should be avoided** if you have cancer. Not more than 60 grams of protein per day(1 gm per kg body weight) is needed normally. Only one type of protein should be consumed per meal so as to avoid stress on the digestive organ. Don't take animal protein such as beef during the evening meal because our digestive system is less active at night and excessive proteins not broken down can result in toxicity and the promotion of cancer. Organic meat should be chosen over commercially raised meat. The best beef comes from grass-fed cattle, and the best chicken are free-range organically

fed poultry. Avoid most dairy products except organic yogurt, organic buttermilk and organic low-fat cottage cheese.
- Take more vegetable proteins such as lentils, chickpeas, kidney beans, lima beans and green peas.
- Raw almonds are excellent sources of protein for cancer patients. It can also be ground to make almond butter. Peanuts must be avoided for their possible aflatoxin contamination. Seeds such as sesame, pumpkin and sunflower should be eaten raw.

Dietary Principles for Easy Digestion

1. Easy to digest food include:

- Spouted beans
- Grains with vegetables
- Vegetables with medium starch content such as carrot, parsnip, squash, pumpkin and corn.
- Medium-starch food mixed with high-starch foods such as cereals, potato, rice, sweet potato and yam.

2. Moderately easy to digest food includes

- Proteins with leafy green vegetables.

3. Difficult to digest food includes

- Proteins with starch food.
- Oil with protein.
- Fruits with vegetables.
- Proteins with sweet fruits such as papayas, bananas and figs.
- Acidic fruits such as grapefruits, lemons, limes, oranges, all berries, tomatoes, and cucumber).
- Sub-acid fruits such as apples, apricots, mangoes, nectarines, peaches, grapes and raisins.

Do I Have to be a Vegetarian?

You have to decide this for yourself. Basically, **it is not necessary to be a total vegetarian,** although we all know that the vegetarian diet is very healthy and ideal for fighting cancer. If we are regular meat eaters, it will be very difficult for us to change overnight. We may perhaps take small amounts of meat for a start and then gradually reduce this amount. For example, those of Nordic-Germanic ancestry have the constitution to use meat and dairy products well, but have difficulty with large quantities of plant-based protein such as soy.

Many people will find a sudden switch of diet very stressful. As such, a **drastic change in diet is not favorable.** It will probably lead to more stress. We should take our time to change our diet. Sometimes, this period can be as long as one to two years, but the change should definitely not be attempted within one to two weeks.

Whey Protein to Supplement Nutrition

Cancer uses energy in the most inefficient way. The majority of the cancer patients die of cachexia. This happens because the body has not enough nutrition to maintain the greedy appetite of the cancer cells. The cancer process exhausts all the energy reserves in these cancer patients. The loss of reserves is often not replenished due to the patient's poor appetite. It is therefore very important for a cancer patient to have a balanced and easily assimilated high-energy diet. Their diet should consist of whole grains, leafy vegetables, legumes and low-glycemic fruits. Whey protein has long been a source of protein for many countries. It is now considered an excellent protein supplement.

To compare protein sources we use an index called the Biological Value. The biological value indicates the quality level of proteins. It is a measure of how easily the body can use the particular protein.

This is often reflected as a percentage. Biological values tell us which proteins are best at aiding nitrogen retention in muscles. The biological value of whey protein is higher than that of milk, fish, beef, soy, wheat, beans and peanuts.

Whey proteins retain the highest amount of immune-enhancing proteins. These include:

- Lactoferrin, an iron-binding, iron-modulating protein that has anti-viral, antibacterial and anti-inflammatory properties.
- Immunoglobulins that support the immune system.
- Lactoferrin and immunoglobulins provide generous amounts of cysteine and glutamine. These are precursors to glutathione, the body's main antioxidant. It provides intracellular defense against oxidative stresses caused by free radicals, reactive oxygen intermediates and toxic chemicals.

Studies have indicated that whey proteins have anti-cancer properties. During a study conducted, six prostate cancer patients who were given whey proteins experienced anti-cancer effects. It was also concluded that whey protein at 20 to 30 grams daily reduced the PSA (a marker for prostatic cancer) concentrations. However, no firm conclusion was drawn and more thorough studies will have to be carried out.

But note that although whey protein is a good source for supplementation, it cannot be used as a meal replacement.

HOW FOOD-BASED ANTIOXIDANTS FIGHT CANCER

We will now look at how food with antioxidant properties fights cancer.

Phase 1 (Initiation Phase)

In this phase, enzymes are produced to break down pro-carcinogens to carcinogens. Garlic and onions limit the production of phase-1 enzymes.

Phase 2 (Promotion Phase)

Enzymes are produced to remove residuals left behind by the phase-1 enzymes. Broccoli helps to boosts production of phase-2 enzymes.

Cell promotion leads to uncontrolled cell growth. Flaxseed and fish oil stop cell growth. The hormone estrogen promotes cell growth. The consumption of soy products will compete with estrogen cell receptors and reduce cancer formation.

Phase 3 (Angiogenesis)

Cancer cell spreads by creating new blood vessels. Red grapes help to prevent the development of new blood vessels via their enzyme called co-oxygenase 2 (or cox 2) inhibitors.

SPECIFIC ANTI-CANCER FOODS

As explained in the previous paragraph, the growth cycle of cancer cells involves various phases. We will now take a closer look at some of those anti-cancerous foods mentioned there.

Carotenoids

This is a group of more than 500 different pigments found in plants. They include beta-carotene found in carrots, leutin and lycopene found in tomatoes and zeaxanthin. They perform a slightly different function from other antioxidants. Certain forms of carotenoids can destroy singlet oxygen, which is bad oxygen. Studies have shown that diets rich in carotenoids can reduce cancer.

Cruciferous vegetables

Good examples are broccoli, cauliflower, Brussels sprouts and bok choy. They produce phytoestrogen, which acts as an estrogen competitor and reduces the amount of estrogen responsible for promoting breast, cervical, ovarian and uterine cancer.

Laetrile (amyglalin)

Laetrile is a chemical found in the kernels of apricot pits, apple seeds, bitter almonds and some stone fruits and nuts. Some laetrile promoters call it vitamin B17.
Some researchers believe that laetrile can improve the patient's sense of well-being, relieve the pain of cancer and reduce pain caused by medication.

Laetrile is broken down into glucose, benzaldehyde and cyanide. These three components help to give the patients extra energy and reduce their pain. Cyanide destroys cancer cells. When laetrile is used together with vitamin A and enzymes, its anti-cancer effects are even more pronounced.

The recommended dosage is 9 gram intravenously daily for up to three weeks, followed by 500 mg three times daily by mouth. The patient should continue to take this supplement even during remission according some physicians. Eating two to four apricot kernels two to three times a day will also provide the recommended amount. Unsulfured dried fruits are also excellent. Blackberries, raspberries, cranberries, gooseberries and elderberries can also be substituted.

Laetrile is ineffective against brain cancers, sarcomas of the muscle, connective tissues, fat tissues and bone tissues. It is useful for cancers of the lungs, breasts, colon, ovaries, stomach, esophagus and the prostate and lymphomas.

Many doctors are skeptical about laetrile, and the laetrile controversy goes back some 50 years and is still raging. It is not available in the USA. Some physicans believe that laetrile causes cyanide poisoning. However, this apparently only occurs when laetrile is taken orally when it is broken down to cyanide. The safe procedure is to inject laetrile intravenously as this method does not release any cyanide.

Garlic

Garlic has been used since biblical times as an immune booster and antibacterial agent. It can stimulate the immune system and is a natural antibiotic and antioxidant. **Garlic eaters have lower risk of throat, stomach and colon cancer.**

Raw garlic taken orally is the most effective but it can be quite difficult to swallow because of its pungent smell. Cooked garlic is not as effective as cooking destroys its antioxidant properties. An alternative is the tablet or capsule form, which can be taken once or twice a day.

Some Special Considerations

- Gingko biloba extract should be taken for one month after radiation therapy. It helps to cleanse the blood and enhances circulation. The recommended dosage is 100mg a day.
- Sea vegetables are excellent for thyroid support for at least one month after radiation.

CHAPTER ELEVEN

OTHER NATURAL THERAPIES

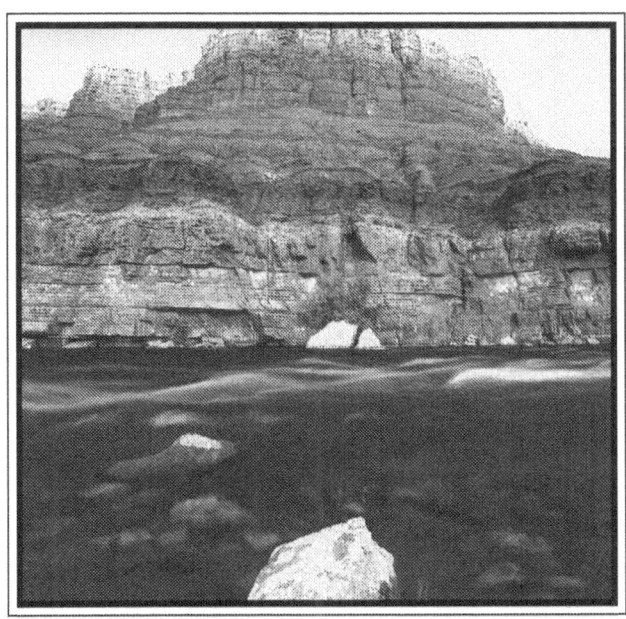

"It amazes me how much of what passes for knowledge
in cancer therapy turns out to be incomplete,
inadequate, and anecdotal."

Ralph Moss, PhD Noted Cancer Researcher in
The Cancer Industry.

In the last few chapters, we have looked at ways of treating cancer by consuming non-toxic food-based natural compounds. We are now very clear that these natural compounds can be used to boost our immunity, stop cancer growth, optimize intracellular functions, maintain a healthy biological terrain and detoxify our bodies.

In this final chapter, we will examine other forms of natural therapies not related to natural compounds but related to the characteristics of the cancerous process.

Many of these therapies have been extensively clinically used for decades. Scientific documentation and double blind studies required by modern medicine are incomplete, but anecdotal reports from patients point to their validity. Suffice to say that provided there is no harm, many patients, out of desperation, will attempt to implement any one or all of these modalities. Many advance cancer clinics in Mexico or Western Europe employ these modalities. They are by no means "quackery" as others may wish you to believe. It is fair to say, however, that there is simply not enough data to pass the high level of scientific scrutiny.

Hyperthermia to Kill Cancer Cells

Hyperthermia uses concentrated therapeutic heat to treat cancer. The therapy works on the basis that cancer cells are far more sensitive to heat than healthy cells. When the cancer cells are heated, their enzymes, membranes and DNA are damaged and their blood supply will be cut off, resulting in the eventual death of the cancer cells.

There are five different methods of achieving hyperthermia.

1. Firstly, the body temperature of the patient is raised to 103°F using sauna-like chambers.

2. Secondly, heat is only directed at the tumor or metastasized sites. In this case, the temperature is raised to a high of between 107°F and 109.4°F.
3. In the third method, direct strong infrared radiation is applied to the cancerous areas. Probes or focused emitting devices are used in these methods.
4. The next method is to raise the whole-body temperature in a more moderate way, from 98.6°F to 104°F using whole-body wet wraps, saunas and hot baths.
5. The final method involves removing blood from the body and cycling it through a heat machine. As such, the temperature of the blood is raised and then reinfused into the body.

During the hyperthermia treatment, ginseng and quercetin should be taken to enhance the effectiveness of the treatment. Quercetin helps to stop histamine release and synthesis of proteins that help tumors resist heat stresses. It also prevents the transport of lactic acid out from the cancer cell. The acidity of the cancer cell is reduced, preventing cancer growth.

Whether or not this treatment is successful depends on the site and stage of the cancer, the age of patient, immune resistance and the tumor response rate. This treatment is very popular in Europe.

Bioresonance to Induce Cell Decomposition (Lysis)

This method uses computerized equipment to irradiate patients with energy in the form of sound frequencies. Some people refer to this as Rife Technology as it was first advanced by Dr Rife. The energy emitted into our bodies must match the vibratory frequencies of elements within our bodies. This mechanism radiates energy with their aggregate thus allowing the atoms in the cell to create a signature oscillation pattern. As cancer cells and normal cells have different vibratory frequencies, radio waves are set to resonate with these frequencies. The targeted cancer cells are then destroyed.

Some doctors have used this therapy for many decades. However, its applications and effectiveness are still very controversial due to the lack of scientific research and clinical studies.

Ultraviolet Blood Irradiation (UBI) Therapy

This therapy is also called photoluminotescence. It involves exposing small quantities of the cancer patient's blood to ultraviolet light so as to stimulate and boost the immune system and destroy cancer cells.

During this procedure, a small amount of blood is removed from the body. After irradiating this blood with ultraviolet light, it is returned intravenously to the patient. This procedure may be done daily and it generally takes one to two hours. This therapy can inactivate toxins, destroy and inhibit bacteria and viruses, increase the oxygen levels in the blood and decrease platelet aggregation.

Oxygenating Therapies

Cancer cells and oxygen do not go together. Cancer cells cannot live well in an oxygen-rich environment.

Oxygen therapy also boosts the immune system and various enzyme systems by increasing the production of cytokines. These are immunologically active proteins that directly and indirectly destroy microorganisms or tumor cells.

Oxygen can be introduced into the body by a variety of mechanisms.

- **Hyperbaric oxygen chamber.** Oxygen is forced into the body via a pressurized chamber. This process enriches the oxygen content in the body or cell.
- **Aerobic exercise** gives oxygen to the entire body system.
- **Ozone insuflation** via the ear, rectum or by ozoning the patient's blood can increase oxygen in the body. Ozone, a less stable form of oxygen, contains three oxygen atoms per molecule. It is more

reactive than oxygen and readily oxidizes other chemicals. When the extra oxygen atom breaks away, the O_2 molecule is left behind. The net effect is an increase in the body's oxygen level. Ozone therapy can be combined with a proper diet, nutritional supplementations, herbs, botanicals and other natural non-toxic cancer therapies for maximum effectiveness.

- **Autohemotherapy.** This is a simple procedure whereby 100 to 250 ml of the patient's blood is removed and then mixed with ozone and oxygen. Thereafter, it is reinfused into the patient's bloodstream. The entire process takes about 45 minutes. It is the most common form of ozone therapy today and very safe.
- **Germanium Sesquioxide.** This natural element helps the body activate and use oxygen. It is administered intravenously or orally. The dose is 500 mg a day during initial therapy. It can be taken orally at 100 to 150 mg a day.
- **Hydrogen Peroxide Infusion Therapy.** This therapy has been very successful and can be used on its own or together with chemotherapeutic agents. It can increase the body's immune response and make cancer cells more sensitive to the effects of radiation therapy. Using hydrogen peroxide diluted in water can increase the oxygen level in the tumor area and help to destroy it. In the Hospital Santa Monica, more than 30,000 infusions were administered. There was no reported negative reaction. The infusion for the cancer patient is slow over a period of 1 to 1.5 hours. After that, they reported improved mental clarity and a sense of relaxation. We need to flush our bodies with lots of antioxidants when this method is used. As such, the hydrogen peroxide infusion is often alternated with intravenous vitamin C drips.

Magnetic Therapy

The basis of magnetic therapy is simple. In our bodies are magnetic fields that are generated by the chemical reactions within the cells and the ionic currents of the nervous system. The catalytic reactions of enzymes are all driven by magnetic fields and produce magnetic field themselves. Each cell is a small magnet and the whole body is a gigantic magnet with a low magnetic field force.

Today, scientists have found that external magnetic fields can affect the body's function. This therapy restores the body's healthy magnetic fields and promotes recovery from cancer. It works on the notion that when the north magnetic pole is applied to a cancer growth or an area of inflammation, the cancer growth will be inhibited. On the other hand, the south pole tends to stimulate cancer growth.

Studies showed that when tissue culture was exposed to both positive and negative magnetic fields, the cancer receded in an environment of negative field. On the other hand, when a positive magnetic field was applied, the cancer grew. As such, some scientists are looking to test the notion that negative polarity magnetic fields have beneficial effect on living organisms whereas positive polarity magnetic fields have a bad effect.

There are no known side effects in this therapy. It has been implied that a negative electric field maintains the alkaline state, thus preventing cancer growth, however more research is needed.

Lymphatic Therapy

Lymphatic therapy enhances the immune system's ability for phagocytosis of the metastatic cancer cell. It also increases the negative charges present on the wall of the fluid system, thus destroying cancer cells. This therapy involves opening drainage sites in the upper chest and neck. When the drainage system is opened, lymph is then drained into the bloodstream where it is then channeled to the liver where detoxification occurs.

Commonly, lymphatic therapy employs a special light beam generator that looks like a flashlight. When placed on the body, it opens up the lymphatic drainage system. This process is painless and non-invasive. The lymphatic sessions usually last for 30 to 45 minutes.

Insulin Potentiation Therapy

Since 1928, insulin has been used to treat diabetes in many parts of the world. In 1950, it was also used to treat patients with mental illness. As some of these mental patients also had cancer at the same time, doctors unexpectedly discovered that this insulin therapy cured both their mental condition as well as their cancer.

The reason is logical. Cancer cells thrive on sugar and they have more insulin receptors compared to normal cells. Depriving the cancer cell of sugar is a death warrant for them.

During insulin therapy, the blood sugar level is significantly reduced to 50 mg/dl. At this level, the patient may feel drowsy and weak for a short period when the cancer cells are crying out for sugar. The cancer cell, striving for sugar, takes up sugar rapidly after being starved. Any chemotherapeutic agents, when infused with sugar infusion, will be selectively taken up by the starved cancer cells. This is an effective way to deliver chemotherapeutic agents to target cancer cells without negative effects to normal cells.

Zoetron Therapy

This therapy uses a special device called a Zoetron that generates a pulsed magnetic field to create hyperthermia directed only at cancerous cells. Normal cells are not damaged and there are no adverse side effects in this treatment.

Specifically the Zoetron device delivers a magnetic field in the form of vibrations to heat up particles in the cancer cells. As cancer cells contain a higher concentration of iron than normal cells, they are more attracted to the magnetic pulse. Vibration energy is transformed into heat and cancer cells are killed when the heat becomes intense. The temperature threshold for cancer cell death is 42°C to 43°C.

This therapy is practiced in Mexico. A normal course of treatment consists of 30 sessions lasting two hours each. Studies have shown that this treatment is very effective in prolonging the lives of pancreatic cancer patients.

EPILOG

By now, we know that cancer is not simply the localized lumps and bumps that we have been programmed to accept through the years. Cancer in the adult can often be viewed as a degenerative process with symptoms representative of underlying systemic dysfunction. We all have cancer cells in our bodies. It is only when our body is unable to get rid of the cancer cells that a disease process takes place. This is when we are diagnosed as having cancer.

What are the underlying system's dysfunctions? There are many factors, including emotional, diet, drugs and chemicals, infections, genetic mutation and environmental pollutants.

Conventional treatments look at cancer as a disease state. The natural-oriented doctor views cancer as a set of symptoms reflecting underlying disease.

The conventional treatment of surgery, radiation and chemotherapy has been the cornerstone of cancer treatment over the past 50 years. Today, the clinical success of these treatments has reached a plateau. There is an urgent need to rise above this cure plateau by trying fresh approaches.

In the United States, much controversy has arisen between mainstream and alternative medicine. The cancer establishment, championed by the American Cancer Society (ACS) has characterized natural and adjunctive cancer therapies as the works of quacks preying on desperate and credulous cancer victims, while the proponents of alternative therapies have depicted established therapies as the "cut, burn, and poison" therapies of a cynical and profit-driven conspiracy.

Interestingly, this adversarial position has disappeared in many European countries like Switzerland, Germany, England and the Netherlands, where an open co-existence of natural and conventional medicine in a complementary setting prospers. Many treatments not available in the United States are widely available and practiced legally in these countries. Looking at vitality statistics, these countries also rank ahead of the United States in longevity.

Natural-oriented doctors view natural therapies as a way to complement conventional therapies and help the patient overcome cancer without toxic side effects. After reading this book, you should realize that both conventional and alternative therapies are effective forms of cancer treatment. Today, many natural and non-toxic modalities are offered in many countries such as Switzerland, Germany, England, Mexico and the Netherlands. The results are excellent. However, in the United States, it is still not well recognized. Many doctors do not recommend them. The most common reasons are ignorance and rigid medical standards. This may be the underlying reason as to why United States ranks a low 13th on the longevity scale despite having the most advance medical technology in the world.

In the words of John Diamond, MD, & Lee Cowden, MD:

Conventional cancer treatments are in place as the law of the land because they pay, not heal, the best.

Modern natural medicine approaches cancer therapy by incorporating the use of antioxidants, lifestyle changes, herbs, and dietary modification to beat it. These approaches will also help to prepare the cancer patient's body for conventional treatment. The side effects will be reduced. Neither conventional nor alternative treatment holds the magic bullet in cancer treatment. Combining the best of both worlds to beat cancer makes the most logical sense for the patient.

Looking into the future, the good news is that less toxic and target-specific chemotherapeutic agents are being developed. More research and clinical studies are also being conducted on natural therapies. The general success rates are getting higher when both conventional alternate treatments are used. However, we must also note that just as there are conventional therapies that do not work, the same should be expected of certain natural or alternative therapies. The success of a treatment often depends on the stage of cancer, the age, the immunity status, and the tumor response rate of the patient.

As more research is carried out new cures will be found. Unfortunately, most cancer patients do not have time to wait. Sometimes, they are only given a few more months to live. They and their families are desperate and will look for any modality that offers a promise. This book has attempted to put into a logical framework the hundreds of alternative options available so we can further discuss them with our doctor.

Practitioners of natural therapies range from lay people with no medical training to highly trained doctors who have departed from their mainstream practice. The vast majority are doctors seeking to supplement careful use of conventional therapies with natural approaches and not to replace them.

The complete natural healing program should include a therapeutic blend of vitamins, herbs, minerals and enzymes. Choosing the proper combination and dosage of these natural compounds is an important key to success. This comes with not only experience but also an extensive medical knowledge of the cancer disease. It is therefore highly recommended to consult a nutritionally oriented physician with an orthomolecular oncology experience before you start any treatment program.

REFERENCES

Abou-Issa H et al: Relative efficacy of glucarate on the initiation and promotion phase of rate mammary carcinogenesis. *Anticancer Res* 1995;May-Jun:15(3):805-10.

Abou-Issa HM. et al: Putative metabolites derived from dietary combinations of calcium glucarate and N-(4-hydroxyphenyl) retinamide act synergistically to inhibit the induction of rat mammary tumors by 7,12-dimethylbenz(a) anthracene. *Proc Natl Acad Sci USA* 85(12):4181-4, Jun 1988.

Ahmad N, Adhami VM, Afaq F, Feyes DK, Mukhtar H. Resveratrol causes WAF-1/p21-mediated G(1)-phase arrest of cell cycle and induction of apoptosis in human epidermoid carcinoma A431 cells. *Clin Cancer Res.* 2001 May;7(5):1466-73.

Aidoo A, Lyn-Cook LE, Lensing S, Wamer W: Ascorbic acid (vitamin C) modulates the mutagenic effects produced by an alkylating agent in vivo. *Environ Mol Mutagen* 24:220-228, 1994.

Ames BN et al: Oxidants, antioxidants, and the degenerative diseases of aging. *Proc Natl Acad Sci USA* 90(17):7915-22, 1993.

Anonymous: Toxicologic Consequences of Oral Aluminium. *Nutrition Reviews* 45: 72-4, 1987.

Asano K. et al: Production of hydrogen peroxide in cancerous tissue by intravenous administration of sodium 5,6-benzylidene-L-ascorbate. *Anticancer Research* 19(1A): 229-36, Jan-Feb 1999.

Balch J, Balch P. *Prescription for Nutritional Healing.* 2nd Edition. Avery Publishing Group, New York.

Ballatori N, Clarkson TW: Dependence of Biliary Excretion of Inorganic Mercury on the Biliary Transport of Glutathione. *Biochem Pharmacol* 33:1093-8,1984.

Benade L, Howard T, Burk D. Synergistic killing of Ehrlich ascites carcinoma cells by ascorbate and 3-amino-1,2,4,-triazole. *Oncology* 1969;23:33-43.

Bliznakov E, Casey A, Premuzic E: Coenzymes Q: stimulants of the phagocytic activity in rats and immune response in mice. *Experientia* 26(9): 253-254, 1970.Bussey HJ, DeCosse JJ,

Boari C, et al: Occupational Toxic Liver Diseases: Therapeutic Effects of Silymarin. *Min Med* 72: 2679-88,1985.

Boik J. *Natural Compound in Cancer Therapy.* 2001. Oregon Medical Press, Princeton, Mn.

Boros LG, Bassilian S, Lim S, Lee WN. Genistein inhibits nonoxidative ribose synthesis in MIA pancreatic adenocarcinoma cells: a new mechanism of controlling tumor growth. *Pancreas.* 2001 Jan;22(1):1-7.

Bounous G. Whey protein concentrate (WPC) and glutathione modulation in cancer treatment. *Anticancer Res.* 2000 Nov-Dec;20(6C):4785-92.

Burman, N.D., Parsons, F.M. Hyperalimentation in the treatment of advanced carcinoma with induced magnesium and potassium depletion. *S.A. Med.* Tydskrif. 1976; Oct 2:1695-1702.

Bushman JL. Green tea and cancer in humans: a review of the literature. *Nutr Cancer* 1998;31:151-159.

Cameron E, Campbell A: The orthomolecular treatment of cancer. II. Clinical trial of high-dose ascorbic acid supplements in advanced human cancer. *Chem-Biol Interactions* 9:285-315, 1974.

Cameron E, Pauling L: Ascorbic acid and the glycosaminoglycans. *Oncology* 27:181-192, 1973.

Cameron E, Pauling L: *Cancer and Vitamin C.* New York, (New York: W.W. Norton & Company, Inc, 1979).

Cameron E, Pauling L: Supplemental ascorbate in the supportive treatment of cancer: Prolongation of survival times in terminal human cancer. *Proc Natl Acad Sci* 73:3685-3689, 1976.

Cameron E, Pauling L: Supplemental ascorbate in the supportive treatment of cancer: Reevaluation of prolongation of survival times in terminal human cancer. *Proc Natl Acad Sci* 75:4538-4542, 1978.

Cameron E: Protocol for the use of Vitamin C in the treatment of cancer. *Med Hypoth* 36:190-194, 1991.

Canini F, Bartolucci E, Cristallini, et al: Use of Silymarin in the Treatment of Alcoholic Hepatic Steatosis. *Clin Ter* 114:307-14, 1985.

Carlson J. Reishi Mushroom. *New Editions Health World,* 23-25, April, 1996.

Carter, JP, Macrobiotic diet and cancer survival, *J Amer Coll Nutr,* 12:3:209-215, 1993

Cha CW: A Study on the Effect of Garlic to the Heavy Metal Poisoning of Rat. *J Korean Med Sci* 2:213-23, 1987.

Chen, Chi-Ling, et al. Hormone replacement therapy in relation to breast cancer. *Journal of the American Medical Association,* Vol. 287, February 13, 2002, pp. 734-41.

Chinery R, Brockman JA, Peeler MO, et al. Antioxidants enhances the cytotoxicity of chemotherapeutic agents in colorectal cancer: a p53-independent induction of p21 via C/EBP-beta. *Nat Med* 1997;3;1233-1241

Chow HH, Cai Y, Alberts DS, et al. Phase I pharmacokinetic study of tea polyphenols following single-dose administration of epigallocatechin gallate and polyphenon E. *Cancer Epidemiol Biomarkers Prev.* 2001 Jan;10(1):53-8.

Cohen M, Bhagavan HN: Ascorbic acid and gastrointestinal cancer. *J Am Coll Nutr* 14:565-578, 1995.

Collery, P., Anghileri, L.J., Coudoux, P., Durlach, J. (Magnesium and cancer: Clinical data.) *Magnesium Bull.* 1981; 3:11-20. Complementary treatments highlighted at recent meeting. *Oncology* (Huntington NY) 13(2):166, 1999.

Cortes EP, Gupta M, Chou C, et al.: Adriamycin cardiotoxicity: early detection by systolic time interval and possible prevention by coenzyme Q10. *Cancer Treatment Reports* 62(6):887-891, 1978.

Crane FL, Sun IL, Sun EE: The essential functions of coenzyme Q. *Clinical Investigator* 71(suppl 8):S55-S59, 1993.

Cruess WV, and Alsberg CL, The bitter glucoside of the olive. *J Amer. Chem. Soc.* 1934; 56:2115-7.

Curley RW et al: Activity of D-glucarate analogues: synergistic antiproliferatie effects with retinoid in cultured human mammary tumor cells appear to specifically require the D-glucarate structure. *Life Sci* 1994;54(18):1299-303.

Currier NL, Miller SC. Echinacea purpurea and melatonin augment natural-killer cells in leukemic mice and prolong life span. *J Altern Complement Med.* 2001 Jun;7(3):241-51.

David Marshall, OD, PhD. *Current Concepts on Whey Protein Usage,* Prepared for The Cleveland Eye Clinic.

De Santi C, Pietrabissa A, Spisni R, Mosca F, Pacifici GM. Sulphation of resveratrol, a natural compound present in wine, and its inhibition by natural flavonoids. *Xenobiotica.* 2000 Sep; 30(9):857-66.

Deschner EE, et al: A randomized trial of ascorbic acid in polyposis coli. *Cancer* 50:1434-1439, 1982.

Diamond W, Cowden W. *Definitive Guide to Cancer.* Future Medicine Publishing, Inc. Tiburon Ca. 1997

Di Bella L, Rossi MT: Abstract from Symposium on Melatonin and Pineal Gland. A satellite Symposium of the 8th International Congress of Endocrinology. Hong Kong 1988.

Drewa G, Wozqak A, Palgan K, et al. Influence of quercetin on B16 melanotic melanoma growth in C57BL/6 mice and on activity of some acid hydrolases in melanoma tissue. *Neoplasma.* 2001;48(1):12-8.

Dumitrescu C, Belgun M, Olinescu R, et al: Effect of vitamin administration on the ratio between the pro- and antioxidative factors. *Rom J Endocrinol* 31:81-84, 1993.

Dyke GW, Craven JL, Hall R, Garner RC: Effect of vitamin C supplementation on gastric mucosal DNA damage. *Carcinogenesis* 15:291-295, 1994.

Fearon ER, Vogelstein B: *Tumor suppressor and DNA repair gene defects in human cancer.* In Holland JF and others. Cancer Medicine, Fourth Edition. (Baltimore: Williams & Wilkins, 1997), pp 103-104.

Ferenci P, et al: Randomized Controlled Trial of Silymarin Treatment in Patients with Cirrhosis of the Liver. *J Hepatol* 9:105-13, 1989.

Flora, S.J.S., et al., "Protective Role of Trace Metals in Lead Intoxication," *Toxicology Letters 13* (1982): 51-6.

Folkers K, Brown R, Judy W, Morita M. Survival of cancer patients on therapy with coenzyme Q10. *Biochem Biophys Res Comm* 1993;192:241-245.

Folkers K, Osterborg A, Nylander M, et al: Activities of vitamin Q10 in animal models and a serious deficiency in patients with cancer. *Biochemical and Biophysical Research Communications* 234(2):296-299, 1997.

Folkers K, Porter TH, Bertino JR, et al: Inhibition of two human tumor cell lines by antimetabolites of coenzyme Q10. *Research Communications in Chemical Pathology and Pharmacology* 19(3):485-490, 1978.

Folkers K, Shizukuishi S, Takemura K, et al: Increase in levels of IgG in serum of patients treated with coenzyme Q10. *Research Communications in Chemical Pathology and Pharmacology* 38(2):335-338, 1982.

Folkers K: The potential of coenzyme Q10 (NSC-140865) in cancer treatment. *Cancer Chemotherapy Reports* 4(4):19-22, 1974.

Folkers K, Wolaniuk A: Research on coenzyme Q10 in clinical medicine and in immunomodulation. Drugs Under Experimental and *Clinical Research* XI(8):539-545, 1985.

Folkman, J. 1971. NEJM 285:1182.

Folkman, J. 1976. Isolation of a cartilage factor that inhibits tumor neovascularization. *Science.* 193:70-71.

Folkman, J. abd Klagsburn, M. 1987. Angiogenic factors. *Science.* 235:442-447.

Folkman, J. et al. 1963. *Cancer* 16:453.

Foster, HD,. Lifestyle influences on cancer regression, *Int J Biosoc Res,* 10:1:17-20

Gerson M. *A Cancer Therapy.* 6th Edition. Gerson Institute, Bonita, Ca.

Gerstner BG, Huff JE: Clinical Toxicology of Mercury. *J Toxicol Environ Health* 2:471-526, 1977.

Gey KF. Vitamins E plus C interacting co-nutrients required for optimal health. *Biofactors* 7(1-2):113-74, 1998.

Greco AM, Gentile M, Di Filippo O, Coppola A: Study of blood vitamin C in lung and bladder cancer patients before and after treatment with ascorbic acid. A preliminary report. *Acta Vitaminol Enzymol* 4:155-162, 1982.

Griffin, GE. *World Without Cancer.* 2nd Edition. American Media, Westlake Village, Ca. 1997.

Guenther, T. Functional compartmentation of intracellular magnesium. *Magnesium* 1986; 5:53-59.

Halpern, George.MD, PHD, *Cordyceps, China's healing Mushroom.* Avery Publishing Group, Garden City Parks, NY, 1999. ISBN: 0-89529-811

Hass, G.M., Laing, G.H., Galt, R.M., McCreary, P.A. Recent advances: immunopathology of magnesium deficiency in rats: induction of tumors; incidence, transmission and prevention of lymphoma-leukemia. *Magnesium Bull.* 1981; 3:217-228.

Heerdt AS et al: Calcium Glucarate as a chemo-preventive agent in breast cancer. *Isr J Med Sci* 1995;31(2-3):101-5.

Hennekens CH, Mayrent SL, Willett W. Vitamin A, carotenoids, and retinoids. *Cancer* 1986;58:1837-1841.

Hikino H, et al: Antihepatotoxic Actions of Flavonolignans from Silybum marianum Fruits. *Planta Medica* 50:248-50, 1984.

Hobbs, Christopher. *Medicinal Mushroiom, An Exploration of Tradition, Healing, and Culture*, by L.Ac.,3rd Edition 1996, Interweave Press Inc, Loveland CO. ISBN: 1-884360-01-7.

Hofmann J, Fiebig HH, Winterhalter BR, et al. Enhancement of the antiproliferative activity of cis-diamminedichloroplatinum(II) by quercetin. *Int J Cancer* 1990;45:536-539.

Igura K, Ohta T, Kuroda Y, Kaji K. Resveratrol and quercetin inhibit angiogenesis in vitro. *Cancer Lett.* 2001 Aug 28;171(1):11-6.

Imamura M, Tung T: A Trial of Fasting Cure for PCB Poisoned Patients in Taiwan. *Am J Ind Med* 5:147-53, 1984.

Jaakkola K. et al. Treatemnt with antioxidant and other nutrients in combination with chemotherapy and irradiation in patients with lung cancer. *AnticancerRes* 12, 599-606, 1992.

Jenner A, England TG, Aruoma OI, Halliwell B: Measurement of oxidative DNA damage by gas chromatography-mass spectrometry: ethanethiol prevents artifactual generation of oxidized DNA bases. *Biochem* J 331:365-369, 1998.

Kenneth J. Reishi: Ancient herb for modern times. Sylvan Press, 1992.

Kozuki Y, Miura Y, Yagasaki K. Resveratrol suppresses hepatoma cell invasion independently of its anti-proliferative action. Cancer Lett. 2001 Jun 26;167(2):151-6.

Kurbacher CM, Wagner U, Kolster B, et al. Ascorbic acid (vitamin C) improves the antineoplastic activity of doxorubicin, cisplatin, and paclitaxel in human breast carcinoma cells in vitro. *Cancer Lett* 1996;103:183-189.

Lamm DL, Riggs DR, Shriver JS, et al. Megadose vitamins in bladder cancer: a double-blind clinical trial. *J Urol* 1994;151:21-26.

Larussi D, Auricchio U, Agretto A, et al: Protective effect of coenzyme Q10 on anthracyclines cardiotoxicity: control study in children with acute lymphoblastic leukemia and non-Hodgkin lymphoma. *Molecular Aspects of Medicine* 15(suppl):S207-S212, 1994.

Lazarou J, Pomeranz B, Corey P. Incidence of adverse drug reactions in hospitalized patients. *JAMA.* 1998; 279:1200-1205.

Leape L. Unnecessary surgery. Annu Rev Public Health. 1992; 13:363-383.

Lee, A. and Robert Langer. 1983 Shark cartilage contains inhibitors of tumor angiogenesis. *Science.* 221:1185-1187

Levine M: New concepts in the biology and biochemistry of ascorbic acid. *N Engl J Med* 314:892-902,1986.

Lian F, Li Y, Bhuiyan M, Sarkar FH. P-53-independent apoptosis induced by genestein in lung cancer cells. *Nutr Cancer* 1999;33:125-131.

Lin JM, Lin CC, Chiu HF, Yang JJ, and Lee SG. Evaluation of the anti-inflammatory and liver protective effects of anoectochilus formosanus ganoderma lucidum and gynostemma pentaphyllum in rats. *Am J Chi Med,* 21:59-69, 1993.

"Lingzhi". In Pharmacology and Application of Chinese Materia Medica, Vol. I. Chang HM and But RPH, eds. *World Scientific: Singapore,* 642, 1986.

Lissoni P, Barni S, Ardizzoia A, et al. Randomized study with the pineal hormone melatonin versus supportive care alone in advanced nonsmall cell lung cancer resistant to a first-line chemotherapy containing cisplatin. *Oncology* 1992;49:336-339.

Lissoni P, Barni S, Ardizzoia A, et al. A randomized study with the pineal hormone melatonin versus supportive care alone in patients with brain metastases due to solid neoplasms. *Cancer* 1994;73:699-701.

Lissoni P, Meregalli S, Nosetto L, et al. Increased survival time in brain glioblastomas by a radioneuroendocrine strategy with radiotherapy plus melatonin compared to radiotherapy alone. *Oncology* 1996;53:43-46.

Lissoni P, Paolorossi F, Ardizzoia A. A randomized study of chemotherapy with cisplatin plus etoposide versus chemoendocrine therapy with cisplatin, etoposide and the pineal hormone melatonin as a first-line treatment of advanced non-small cell lung cancer patients in a poor clinical state. *J Pineal Res* 1997;23:15-19.

Lissoni P, Paolorossi F, Tancinin G, et al. A phase II study of tamoxifen plus melatonin in metastatic solid tumor patients. *Br J Cancer* 1996;74:1466-1468.

Liu JF, Lee YW. Vitamin C supplementation restores the impaired vitamin E status of guinea pigs fed oxidized frying oil. *J Nutr* 1998;128(1):116-22.

Lockwood K, Moesgaard S, Folkers K: Partial and complete regression of breast cancer in patients in relation to dosage of coenzyme Q10. Biochemical and *Biophysical Research Communications* 199(3):1504-1508, 1994.

Lockwood K, Moesgaard S, Hanioka T, et al.: Apparent partial remission of breast cancer in "high risk" patients supplemented with nutritional antioxidants, essential fatty acids and coenzyme Q10. *Molecular Aspects of Medicine* 15(suppl):S231-S240, 1994.

Lockwood K, Moesgaard S, Yamamoto T, et al.: *Biochemical and Biophysical Research Communications* 212(1): 172-177, 1995.

Lockwood K, Moesgaard S, Yamamoto T, Folkers K. Progress on therapy of breast cancer with vitamin Q10 and the regression of metastases. *Biochem Biophys* Res Comm 1995;212:172-177.

Lothian, B, Grey, V, Kimoff, J, Lands, LC. Treatment of Obstructive Airway Disease With a Cysteine Donor Protein, *Chest 2000* 117:914-916

Lund EL, Quistorff B, Spang-Thomsen M, Kristjansen PEG. Effect of radiation therapy on small-cell lung cancer is reduced by ubiquinone intake. *Folia Microbiol* 1998;43:505-506.

Maramag C et el: Effect of vitamin C on prostate cancer cells in vitro: effect on cell number, viability, and DNA synthesis. *Prostate* 32(3):188-95, Aug 1, 1997.

McCoy, J.H., Kenney, M.A. *Magnesium and immune function: a review.* In Magnesium in Cellular Processes and Medicine. Eds: B.M. Altura, J. Durlach, M.S. Seelig, Publ. S. Karger, Basel, Switzerland 1987: 196-211.

Miodini P, Fioravanti L, DiFronzo G, Cappelletti V. The two phyto-oestrogens genistein and quercetin exert different effects on oestrogen receptor function. Br J *Cancer* 1999;80:1150-1155.

Moertel CG, Fleming TR, Creagan ET, et al: High-dose vitamin C versus placebo in the treatment of patients with advanced cancer who have had no prior chemotherapy. *N Engl J Med* 312:137-141, 1985.

Morishige F, Murata A: Prolongation of survival times in terminal human cancer by administration of supplemental ascorbate. *J Interntl Acad Prev Med* 5:47-52, 1979.

Moss R. *Cancer Therapy.* Equinox Press Inc., Brooklyn, New York.

Murata A, Morishige F, Yamaguchi H: Prolongation of survival times of terminal cancer patients by administration of large doses of ascorbate. *Int J Vitam Nutr Res Suppl* 23:103-113, 1982.

Murray M, Pizzorno J. *Encyclopedia of Natural Medicine.* 2nd Edition. Prima Health. 1998.

Mortenssson, J., and Meister, A. Glutathione Deficiency Decreases Tissue Ascorbate Levels in Newborn Rats: Ascorbate Spares Glutathione and Protects. *Proc. Natl. Acad. Sci.* USA 88:4656-46460, 1991.

Murakami M, Webb MA: A Morphological and Biochemical Study of the Effects of L-Cysteine on the Renal Uptake and Nephrotoxicity of Cadmium. *Br J Exp Pathol* 62:115-30, 1981.

Myers C, Bonow R, Palmeri S, et al. A randomized controlled trial assessing the prevention of doxorubicin cardiomyopathy by N-acetylcysteine. *Semin Oncol* 1983;10:S53-S55.

Nation JR, et al: Dietary Administration of Nickel: Effects on Behavior and Metallothionein Levels. *Physiol Behavior* 34:349-53, 1985.

Nakagawa H, Yamamoto D, Kiyozuka Y, et al. Effects of genistein and synergistic action in combination with eicosapentaenoic acid on the growth of breast cancer cell lines. *J Cancer Res Clin Oncol.* 2000 Aug;126(8):448-54.

Nielsen M, Ruch RJ, Vang O. Resveratrol reverses tumor-promoter-induced inhibition of gap-junctional intercellular communication. *Biochem Biophys Res Commun.* 2000 Sep 7;275(3):804-9.

Nomura AM, Kolonel LN, Hankin JH, Yoshizawa CN: Dietary factors in cancer of the lower urinary tract. *Int J Cancer* 48:199-205, 1991.

Null G. The Clinician's Handbook of Natural Healing. Kensington Publishing Corp. New York. 1997.

Overvad K, Diamant B, Holm L, et al.: Coenzyme Q10 in health and disease. European *Journal of Clinical Nutrition* 53(10): 764-770, 1999.

Panizzi L et al. The constitution of oleuropein, a bitter glucoside of the olive with hypotensive action. *Gazz. Chim.* Ital; 1960; 90:1449-85.

Parsons, F.M., Edwards, G.F., Anderson, C.K., Ahmad, S., Clark, P.B., Hetherington, C., Young, G.A. Regression of malignant tumours in magnesium and potassium depletion induced by diet and haemodialysis. *Lancet* 1974; 1:243-244.

Passwater RA, Cranton EM: *Trace Elements, Hair Analysis and Nutrition* (New Canaan, CT: Keats, 1983).

Pauling, Linus: *How to live longer and feel better.* (New York: Avon Books)

Pelton R, Overholser L. *Alternatives in Cancer Therapy.* Simon and Schuster, New York. 1994

Pepping J: Coenzyme Q. *Am J of Health-System Phar* 56: 519-521, 1999.

Petkov V and Manolov P. Pharmacological analysis of the iridoid oleuopein. *Drug Res.*, 1972; 22(9); 1476-86.

Phillips D, Christenfeld N, Glynn L. Increase in US medication-error deaths between 1983 and 1993. *Lancet.* 1998; 351:643-644.

Ponz de Leon M, Roncucci L: Chemoprevention of colorectal tumors: role of lactulose and of other agents. *Scand J Gastroenterol Suppl* 222:72-75, 1997.

Prudden, John. 1965. The clinical acceleration of healing with a cartilage preparation: A controlled study. *JAMA.* 192:252.

Prudden, John and Balessa. 1974. The biological activity of bovine cartilage perparations. *Seminars in Arthritis and Rheumatism.* Vol 3 (4):287-320.

Quilin P. Beating Cancer with Nutrition. *Nutritional Times Press,* Calsbad, Ca.

Reddy VG, Khanna N, Singh N. Vitamin C augments chemotherapeutic response of cervical carcinoma HeLa cells by stabilizing P53. *Biochem Biophys Res Commun.* 2001 Mar 30;282(2):409-15.

Reiser S: "Effects of Dietary Sugars on Metabolic Risk Factors Associated with Heart Disease." *Nutritional Health 3,*1985, pp. 203-216

Renis HE, In vitro antiviral activity of calcium elenolate, an antiviral agent. *Antimicrob. AgentsChemother.,* 1970; 167-72.

Riordan NH, Riordan HD, Meng X, et al. Intravenous ascorbate as a tumor cytotoxic chemotherapeutic agent. *Med Hypotheses* 1995;44:207-213.

Rivers JM. Safety of high-level vitamin C ingestion. Ann NY Acad Sci 1988;498:445-454.

Rutter M, Russell-Jones R, et al: *Lead versus Health: Sources and Effects of Low-Level Lead Exposure* (New York: John Wiley, 1983).

Salmi HA, Sarna S: Effect of Silymarin on Chemical, Functional, and Morphological Alteration of the Liver: A Double-Blind Controlled Study. *Scand J Gastroenterol* 17:417-21, 1982.

Sarre H: Experience in the Treatment of Chronic Hepatopathies with Silymarin. *Arzneim-Forsch* 21:1209-12, 1971.

Sauberlich H: Pharmacology of Vitamin C. *Annu Rev Nutr* 14:371-391, 1994.

Schmidt KH, Hagmaier V, Hornig DH, et al: Urinary oxalate excretion after large intakes of ascorbic acid in man. *Am J Clin Nutr* 34:305-311, 1981.

Schwartz JA, Liu G, Brooks SC. Genistein-mediated attenuation of tamoxifen-induced antagonism from estrogen receptor-regulated genes. *Bioch Biophys Res Comm* 1998;253:38-43.

Seeley S: Diet and breast cancer: the possible connection with sugar consumption. *Med Hypotheses* 11(3):319-27, Jul 1983.

Seelig, M.S. The requirement of magnesium by the normal adult. *Am. J. Clin. Nutr.* 1964; 14:342-390.

Seifter E, Rettura G, Padawer J. Vitamin A and beta-carotene as adjunctive therapy to tumour excision, radiation therapy and chemotherapy. In Prasad K, ed. *Vitamins Nutrition and Cancer.* New York: Karger Press; 1984:2-19.

Setchell KD, Brown NM, Desai P, et al. Bioavailability of pure isoflavones in healthy humans and analysis of commercial soy isoflavone supplements. *J Nutr.* 2001 Apr;131(4 Suppl):1362S-75S.

Shang S et al: Dietary carotenoids and Vitamins A, C, and E and risk of breast cancer. *J Natl Cancer Inst* 1999 Mar 17;91(6):547-56.

Shen F, Xue X, Weber G. Tamoxifen and genistein synergistically down-regulate signal transduction and proliferation in estrogen receptor-negative human breast carcinoma MDA-MB-435 cells. *Anticancer Res* 1999;19:1657-1662.

Shiu SY, Xi SC, Xu JN, et al. Inhibition of malignant trophoblastic cell proliferation in vitro and in vivo by melatonin. *Life Sci.* 2000 Sep 15;67(17):2059-74.

Shklar G, Schwartz J, Trickler D, Reid S. Regression of experimental cancer by oral administration of combined alpha-tocopherol and beta-carotene. *Nutr Cancer* 1989;12:321-325.

Sriganth INP, Premalatha B. Dietary curcumin with cisplatin administration modulates tumour marker indices in experimental fibrosarcoma. *Pharmacol Res* 1999;39:175-179.

Stanislaus CS. Lingzhi Medicine of Kings. *New Editions Health World,* 38-41, June, 1995.

Starfield, B. Journal American Medical Association Vol 284 July 26, 2000.

Stavinoha WB, et al. *Study of the anti-inflammatory activity of Ganoderma lucidum. Presented at the Third Academic/Industry Joint Conference (AIJC),* Sapporo, Japan, 1990.

Steinhausen D, et al: Evaluation of systemic tolerance of 42.0 degrees C infrared-A whole-body hyperthermia in combination with hyperglycemia and hyperoxemia. A Phase-I study. *Strahlenther Onkol* 170(6):322-34, Jun 1994.

Sugiura, K., Benedict, S.R. Influence of magnesium on the growth of carcinoma, sarcoma and melanoma in animals. *Am. J. Cancer* 1935; 23:300- 310.

Support Care Cancer 5(2): 126-29, March 1997. *The Annual Meeting of the American Society for Cell Biology Washington DC* (December 13, 1999).

Unverferth DV, Jagadeesh JM, Unverferth BJ, et al. Attempt to prevent doxorubicin induced acute human myocardial morphologic damage with acetylcysteine. *J Natl Cancer Inst* 1983;71:917-920.

Valcic S et al: Antioxidant chemistry of green tea catechins. *ChemRes Toxicol* 1999;12(4): 382-6.

VandeCreek L, Rogers E, Lester J. Use of alternative therapies among breast cancer outpatients compared with the general population. *Altern Ther Health Med* 1999; 5: 71-76.

Valenzuela A, et al: Selectivity of Silymarin on the Increase of the Glutathione Content in Different Tissues of the Rat. *Planta Med* 55:420-2, 1989.

Veer WLC et al. A Compound isolated from europaea. Recueil,1957; 76:839-40.

Vogel G, et al: Studies on Pharmacodynamics, Site and Mechanism of Action of Silymarin, the Antihepatotoxic Principle from Silybum marianum (L.) Gaer. *Arzneim-Forsch* 25:179-85, 1975.

Volk T, et al. pH in human tumor xenografts: effect of intravenous administration of glucose. *Br J Cancer* 68(3):492-500, Sep 1993.

Von Ardenne M. Principles and concept 1993 of the Systemic Cancer Multistep Therapy (SCMT). Extreme whole-body hyperthermia using the infrared-A technique IRATHERM 2000 — selective thermosensitisation by hyperglycemia-circulatory back-up by adapted hyperoxemia. *Strahlenther Onkol* 170(10):581-9, Oct 1994

Von Oefele F. Some remarks on the treatment of cancerous growths with selenium compounds. *American Medicine* 1912;18:216-219.

Wagdi P, Fluri M, Aeschbacher B, et al. Cardioprotection in patients undergoing chemo- and/or radiotherapy for neoplastic disease. *Jpn Heart J* 1996;37:353-359.

Wagner H: *Antihepatotoxic Flavonoids.* in V. Cody, E. Middleton, and J.B. Harbourne, eds. Plant Flavonoids in Biology and Medicine: Biochemical, Pharmacological, and Structure-Activity Relationships (New York: Alan R. Liss, In., 1986), 545-558.

Walaszek Z et al: Metabolism, uptake, and excretion of a D-glucaric acid salt and its potential use in cancer prevention. *Cancer Detect Prev* 1997;21(2):178-90.

Wasson RG. *Divine mushroom of immortality.* Harcourt, Brace, Jovanovich, Los Angeles, 80-93, 1968.

Weijl NI, Cleton FJ, Osanto S. Free radicals and antioxidants in chemotherapy induced toxicity. *Cancer Treat Rev* 1997;23:209-240.

Weingart SN, Wilson RM, Gibberd RW, Harrison B. Epidemiology and medical error. *BMJ.* 2000; 320:774-777. *World Health Report 2000.* World Health Organization.

Wolter F, Akoglu B, Clausnitzer A, Stein J. Downregulation of the cyclin d1/cdk4 complex occurs during resveratrol-induced cell cycle arrest in colon cancer cell lines. *J Nutr.* 2001 Aug;131(8):2197-203.

Xi SC, Siu SW, Fong SW, Shiu SY. Inhibition of androgen-sensitive LNCaP prostate cancer growth in vivo by melatonin: association of antiproliferative action of the pineal hormone with mt1 receptor protein expression. *Prostate.* 2001 Jan 1;46(1):52-61.

Yost KJ: Cadmium, the Environment and Human Health: An Overview. *Experentia* 40:157-64, 1984.

Zi X, Agarwal R. Silibinin decreases prostate-specific antigen with cell growth inhibition via G1 arrest, leading to differentiation of prostate carcinoma cells: implications for prostate cancer intervention. *Proc Natl Acad Sci* 1999;96:7490-7495.

A

A. annua L, 180
abdominal
   cramps, 175
   pain, 60, 158
ABM, 162, 163
Abram Hoffer, 12, 53, 91,
   124, 151, 220
AbulKalam M. Shamsuddin,
   167
achy joints, 147
acid, 13, 71, 76, 108, 138,
   139, 155, 156, 192, 195,
   226
   acid-forming food, 226
   acidity, 188
   Acid-Producing Foods,
      227
   alpha-linolenic, 230
   ascorbic, 24, 120, 122,
      178
   D-glucaric, 171
   lactic, 75, 76, 83, 189,
      222, 226, 239
   lipoic, 127-130
   panthothenic, 25, 142
   synthetic amino, 215
   urinary uric, 123
acidophilus, 194, 195
acrylamide, 72
acupressure, 99
acupuncture, 99
additive, 201, 226
   chemical, 75
   food, 203, 205
adrenal, 190
   gland, 73, 168
adriamycin, 131
advance-stage
   cancers, 41, 98
adverse reactions, 31
aerobic exercise, 21, 76, 240
aerobic respiration, 76, 137
aflatoxins, 77
agaricus, 25, 164
   Agaricus Blazei Murill,
      162
age-adjusted mortality, 81
agent
   chelating, 23
   chemotherapeutic, 17, 43,
      94, 110, 183, 206, 225,
      241, 243, 246

oral diabetic, 140
age-related
   disease, 36
AIDS, 151, 162
Albert Einstein, 55
Albert Schweitzer, 217
Albert Szent-Gyoergy, 84
alcohol, 38, 132, 154, 168,
   203, 205, 216
alkali, 76
   alkali-forming foods, 226
   alkaline reserves, 190
   alkaline substrates, 226
   alkalinity, 25, 86, 188,
      191, 208
   Alkali-Producing Foods,
      227
   Alkali-Producing
      Vegetables, 227
allergy, 75, 146, 160, 201,
   203, 218
allopathic
   doctors, 34, 99
   medical system, 33, 45
almonds, 191, 231, 235
aloe emodin, 150
aloe vera, 191
alpha lipoic acid complex, 128
alpha-tocopherol, 114
aluminium, 67
American Cancer Society, 37,
   245
American Metabolic Institute,
   16, 90
amino acids, 87, 128, 140,
   161, 178, 192, 195, 202
ammonium salts, 71
Amphotericin B, 141
amygladin, 87
anabolic, 190
anaerobic, 21, 222
   glycolysis, 222
andropause, 36
anemia, 45, 202
angiogenesis, 18, 156, 170,
   174, 177, 234
   induction, 88
   inhibition, 86
animal protein, 230
anise, 208
antacids, 67, 202
anthracycline drug, 137

anti-aging, 86, 113, 135
antibody, 56, 69, 144, 161,
   194, 204
   synthesis, 137
anti-cancer, 11, 17, 25, 48,
   129, 130, 132, 153, 155,
   158, 161, 164-167, 172,
   174, 175, 182, 183, 186,
   219, 221-223, 233-235
anticoagulant, 154
antidepressant drugs, 158
antihistamine, 31
antimony trisulfide, 154
antimycotic, 98
antioxidant
   endogenous, 137
antioxidants, 17, 22, 23, 30,
   87, 89, 90, 95-97, 105-112,
   114, 115, 117, 127,
   129-133, 203, 207, 225,
   226, 234, 235, 241, 246
antiseptic washes, 154
anti-tumor, 95, 96, 149, 150,
   158, 164, 176, 194
antiviral, 98
apathy, 60
apoptosis, 131
apple cider vinegar, 216
apple pectin, 197
apples, 109, 117, 130, 131,
   191, 229, 231
apricots, 191, 229, 231
ARC, 147
arginine, 168
arrhythmia, 31, 141
arsenic, 22, 154, 202, 215
   sulfide, 154
ART, 183-185
artemether, 181, 184, 185
artemisinin, 180-186
   derivatives, 181
   suppositories, 184
arteries, 146
artesunate, 182, 184
arthritis, 39, 107, 146, 160,
   161, 175, 204, 211, 218
artificial sweeteners, 226
asbestos, 69
ascorbate
   deficiency, 118
   induced peroxidation, 119
ascorbyl palmitate, 24, 118,
   178

aspirin, 125, 147
asthma, 149, 161, 168, 203
astragalus, 146
atherosclerosis, 19, 33, 36,
    40, 80, 107
    plaques, 108
auto exhaust, 76
autohemotherapy, 241
auto-immune thyroiditis, 196
azuki beans, 191

B

B-12 destruction, 123
bacteria, 18, 38, 59, 68, 74-76
    144, 147, 148, 150, 166,
    188, 191, 192, 194, 195,
    198, 203, 211, 230, 240
    bacteremia, 147
    bad, 22, 38, 76, 166, 191,
        192, 194, 195
bailey, 223
baking soda, 210
barley grass, 25, 195, 196
base balance, 18, 38
basmati rice, 223, 229
B-Cells, 196
beans, 22, 72, 191, 227, 229,
    231, 233
bee pollen, 191
benign, 180
benzaldehyde, 141
benzene, 69
benzoquinone, 136
beta carotene, 24, 25
beta-glucan, 158, 159, 161,
    164
beta-glucuronidase inhibitor,
    171
beta-sitosterol, 150
bifidobacterium, 195
bile duct, 173
biliary tract cancer, 223
bindweed, 171, 176, 177
bioaccumulation, 66
bioavailability, 161, 184
biochemical, 61, 100
    pathway, 100
bioflavonoids, 109, 130
biological
    Biological Value, 232
    conditions, 15, 81
    terrain, 15, 82, 87, 97,
        100, 188, 192, 238

bioresonance, 239
black box warning, 31
blackberries, 236
blackstrap molasses, 216
bladder habits, 60
blastocystis hominis, 192
blood
    alkalizer, 208, 230
    brain barrier, 184
    clots, 147
    glucose, 223
    poisoning, 147
    purification, 205
    thinners, 125, 147, 156
    vessel, 18, 58, 86, 156,
        166, 170, 172, 174,
        177, 215, 234
bloodroot, 154
bloodstream, 192, 241, 242
blue green algae, 195, 196
B-lymphocytes, 144, 145
body temperature, 18, 155,
    157, 238
bok choy, 208, 225, 235
bone marrow suppression, 44
borage oil, 222
botanical, 87, 241
bovine cartilage, 171, 175,
    176
bovine tracheal cartilage, 175
bowel
    Bowel Tolerance Level,
        123, 124
    movement, 25, 207
    obstructions, 154
BRCA1, 77
breast
    irradiation, 65
    mass, 82
    reconstruction surgery, 77
broccoli, 109, 130, 225,
    227-229, 234, 235
bronchial tree damage, 60
bronchitis, 164
broncho-pneumonia, 127
BTC, 175, 176
BTL, 123, 124
buckthorn bark, 154, 216
buckwheat, 191, 229
buffer salts, 190, 191
bumps, 26, 245
Burdock Root, 149, 152
burn, 9, 14, 44, 53, 245
bursitis, 146

C

cabbage, 191, 208, 230
cachexia, 60, 220, 232
cadmium, 22, 67, 129, 202,
    215
caffeine, 77, 205, 216
    free, 130
calcium, 24, 71, 123, 141,
    142, 149, 154, 171, 174,
    190, 208, 213, 220
    magnesium ratio, 142
    ion, 208
    oxalate, 123
calf liver juice, 218
calories, 22, 109
Cambridge Hospital, 31
cancer, 15, 35
    bladder, 47, 68, 116, 118,
        122
    bone marrow, 30
    brain, 64, 66, 236
    cancerous, 12, 15, 39, 49,
        59, 66, 75, 81, 93, 111,
        112, 117, 118, 200,
        238, 239, 243
    cervical, 60, 74, 126, 139,
        191
    colon, 39, 40
    end-stage, 90, 91
    epithelial cell, 42
    esophageal, 71
    female pancreatic, 46
    forms, 15, 81
    gastric, 74
    gastrointestinal, 60
    hormonal sensitive, 19
    hormone-related, 23
    hospitals, 16, 90
    incidence, 14, 40
    indolent, 59
    inhibitory effect, 86
    kidney, 47
    localized, 57
    male colon, 14, 40
    mammary, 131
    markers, 97
    metastatic, 57, 242
    ovarian, 46, 47, 163, 166,
        218
    pancreatic, 47, 92, 94,
        176, 244
    pathology, 40
    pharyngeal, 68

pro-cancer events, 88
pro-cancerous, 15, 81
rectum, 46
small-cell lung, 91, 96
staging, 56
stomach, 122
terminal, 16, 90, 121, 123, 189
testicular, 42
toolbox, 45
uterine, 47, 125, 235
cancer cell, 11, 15, 17, 18, 21, 22, 26, 36, 41, 43, 45, 57, 58, 60, 61, 72, 77, 81-83, 86, 93-96, 110, 111-114, 116, 117, 119, 126, 128, 131, 133, 136, 140, 150, 154-156, 159, 163, 165, 166, 167, 170, 172, 177-179, 182, 183, 188, 190, 193, 198, 200, 208, 209, 212, 218, 222, 223, 226, 232, 234, 235, 238-245
recurrence, 94
candida albicans, 192
canned food, 67
cantaloupe, 191
capsules, 88, 130, 131, 156, 176
carbohydrate
complex, 21
refined, 71
rich foods, 72
carbon
block, 213
monoxide, 76
tetrachloride, 172
carbonated drinks, 154
carcinogen, 19, 61, 63, 69, 75, 117, 171, 173, 198, 200, 203, 234
chemical, 38
carcinoma, 56, 141, 172
basal cell, 63
renal cell, 176
squamous, 60
transitional cell, 91
cardiac markers, 37
cardiotoxicity, 155
cardiovascular
disease, 35
health, 164
carnitine, 24

carotenoid, 108, 116, 228, 235
carrot, 191, 225, 235
juice, 229
cascara, 154
catabolic, 190
catalase, 108, 119
deficiency, 119
cataract, 107
catechins, 109, 130
caterpillar fungus, 163
cause-and-effect, 78
CBC, 185
cecum, 210
celery, 191, 230
cell
cell-to-cell
communications, 88
decomposition, 239
division, 64, 182
mediated immunity, 140
pre-cancerous, 37, 111
resistance, 95
cellular
energy generation, 17
fatigue, 64
function, 35
mutation, 17
proteins, 39
starvation, 59
terrain, 76
ceramic glazes, 67
cervix, 91, 157
chamomile flower, 216
chelidonine, 165
chemotherapy, 9, 14, 17, 26, 30, 34, 39, 41-45, 48, 50, 59, 82, 83, 85, 93-96, 98, 110, 112, 114, 115, 120, 125, 126, 129-131, 133, 137, 140, 141, 156, 159, 171, 196, 200, 225, 245
cherries, 109, 130
Chester Stock, 150
childhood leukemia, 66
Chinese breathing exercises, 30
chlorella, 25, 195, 196, 197
chloride, 226
chlorinated
swimming pool, 210
water, 68
chlorophyll, 196
choline, 203
chromatin condensation, 172

chromium, 24, 149, 168
chromosomes, 24, 106
chronic, 15, 38-40, 60, 71, 78, 80, 82, 146, 147, 163, 173, 188, 211
degenerative diseases, 38, 40, 80
diarrhea, 60
fatigue, 77, 146, 147, 211
stress, 73
chronic fatigue syndrome, 146
cigarette smoke, 67, 107, 202
cilantro, 208
cirrhosis, 164, 173
cisplatin, 95, 96, 131, 141, 156
citrus
fruits, 109, 117, 130, 131, 230
pectin, 198
Bioflavonoids, 24
cleansing, 206, 216
herbal teas, 216
tea, 216
Clinical Phase of aging, 36
clinically malnourished, 220
closed ecosystem, 18, 76
clostridia, 192
CNS, 182
cocktail, 24, 88, 89, 114, 115
Coenzyme Q10, 25, 89, 127, 136, 137
coffee enemas, 218
cold-water fish, 71, 73
colitis, 154, 210
collagen, 24, 119, 177, 178, 179
collateral damage, 43
colon cleansing, 206, 210, 211
colonic polyps, 122
color, 48, 83, 129, 190
colorectal cancer, 47, 120, 122, 218
computer terminals, 63
computer tomography
scanners, 32
concoctions, 152
constipation, 60, 74, 175, 197, 202, 211
constitution, 232
contaminants, 67, 68
contra-indicated, 112
control group, 91, 114, 120, 121, 223

cooked
  cereal grains, 229
  spinach, 191
co-oxygenase 2, 234
copper, 13, 109
CoQ10, 89, 127, 130, 136, 137-140, 183
cordycep, 163, 164
corn, 71, 166, 176, 222, 231
cortisol, 73, 168
coumadin, 156
cox 2 inhibitors, 234
cranberries, 236
cryptosporidium, 213
cucumber, 191, 208
curcumin, 171, 172
cure plateau, 42, 245
currants, 229
cut, 9, 14, 21, 41, 53, 92, 152, 159, 168, 204, 238, 245
cyanide, 235, 236
cyclo-oxygenase, 132, 173
cytochrome P450 enzyme, 173
cytokines, 145, 156, 240
cytotoxic effect, 95
cytotoxicity, 156

D

dairy foods, 77
damiana leaf, 216
dates, 175, 191
DDT, 65, 66
death, 9, 31, 35, 38, 40, 42, 44, 46, 50, 53, 66, 120, 123, 136, 179, 189, 238, 243, 244
debulking, 41, 81, 92
decaffeinated, 25, 131, 229
degenerative disease, 13, 33, 35, 39, 40
dengue fever, 147
depression, 184, 203, 211
dermal tumor, 118
detoxifying, 18, 23, 25, 30, 41, 75, 86, 87, 92, 94, 97, 100, 117, 171, 172, 186, 194, 197, 200, 201, 203-218, 226, 242
  natural, 218
DHA, 156

diabetes, 19, 33, 36-38, 40, 146, 151, 164, 167, 204, 243
diarrhea, 24, 45, 124, 147, 155, 197
dieldrin, 67
diet, 22, 25, 26, 30, 38, 39, 52, 61, 66, 74, 80, 81, 92, 100, 108, 130, 142, 145, 166, 168, 179, 183, 193, 197, 205, 207, 211, 215-217, 219-223, 228, 229, 232, 241, 245
digestive
  enzymes, 155, 192, 193, 197, 216
  impairment, 73
  tract, 73, 205
Digoxin, 180
DNA, 42, 61, 63, 86, 107, 116, 123, 128, 129, 131, 137, 140, 172, 201, 238
  polymerase B, 131
double-blind data, 85
doxorubicin, 95, 115, 137, 181
drug, 26, 31, 32, 41, 42, 48, 75, 86, 87, 95, 96, 133, 137, 140, 141, 147, 156, 158, 168, 181, 205, 206, 227, 245
  over-the-counter, 67
  statin, 140
dysfunction, 15, 19, 26, 34, 37-39, 52, 59, 81, 99, 245

E

E2, 125
E3, 125
ear, 147, 240
Echinacea, 146, 168
eczema, 150
edema
  scrotum, 176
EDTA, 129, 215
  calcium, 215
  chelation therapy, 129
elderberries, 236
electrical poles, 63
electromagnetism, 38, 61, 77, 99
  electromagnetic fields, 63

electromagnetic radiation, 38, 77
electron, 65, 106, 107, 128
  donor, 128
embryo, 42, 75
EMF, 64
  cumulative exposures, 63
  exposure, 64
emodin, 96
emotional stress, 26, 61, 73
encephalitis, 147
endometrial, 60, 71
endoperoxide bridge, 181
enema, 186, 211
energy, 17, 21, 22, 35, 58-61, 63, 75, 83, 99, 100, 107, 128-130, 135-137, 140, 142, 189, 209, 226, 232, 235, 239, 243
  level, 35, 129, 209
  demanding cells, 137
England, 146, 245, 246
environment, 21, 38, 58, 71, 72, 74-76, 83, 86, 111, 119, 127, 155, 174, 181, 188-190, 192, 202, 205, 208, 212, 220, 222, 226, 228, 240, 242
environmental
  estrogens, 67, 70
  pollutants, 26, 245
  toxins, 17, 67
enzyme, 74, 107, 109, 111, 173, 177, 183, 192, 193, 218, 234, 240
  activator, 218
  enzymatic reactions, 140
  inhibitor, 218
  multi-digestive, 217
  oxidizing, 218
  pancreatic, 74, 183, 186
  phase-2, 234
  proteolytic digestive, 25
  secreting, 18
EPA, 156
epidemic, 67, 70
epsom salt, 210
Epstein-Barr virus, 74, 147
equilibrium, 18
esophagus, 60, 157, 236
ESR, 185
Essiac, 26, 148, 151-153
established protocol, 20, 103
estradiol, 125

estriol, 125
estrogen, 13, 58, 67, 69, 70,
    125, 131, 234, 235
    cell receptors, 234
    receptor positive, 58
excrement, 73, 144, 204,
    207, 208
exercise, 21, 39, 74, 75, 76,
    87, 168, 186, 207, 212,
    216
extracellular,
    serum, 202,
    matrix, 178. 179
extract, 25, 26, 130, 146,
    147, 148, 151, 152, 159,
    160-164, 168, 172, 177,
    203, 236
    glandular, 87
    green tea, 25, 131

F

factory emission, 76
fasting, 206, 207
    complete, 206
fatigue, 60, 176, 189, 202,
    210
fats
    essential, 229
    healthy, 22
    omega-3, 71, 139, 155,
        156, 230
    omega-6, 13, 71, 156
fatty
    infiltration, 173
    streaks, 108
FDA, 31, 42, 43
fecal
    material, 211
    mutagens, 117
fennel, 208
fermentation, 75, 76, 189
fermenting bacteria, 205
ferritin, 185
fertilizers, 226
fetus, 42
fever, 144, 151
fiber, 18, 22, 25, 59, 74, 160,
    165, 192, 196-198, 204,
    207
fibrosis, 97
fibrocystic patient, 125
figs, 191, 231
fish oil, 25, 97, 155, 156, 234

flaxseed, 71, 211, 230
flora, 74, 188, 211
fluoride, 226
    fluoridated water, 68
folic acid, 24, 168, 192
folk medicine, 155, 164
food
    additives, 203, 205
    dyes, 226
foreign bodies, 144
formaldehyde, 203
Fractions A, B, C and D, 159
free radical, 17, 61, 69, 84,
    86, 95, 105-107, 108, 116,
    126, 129, 130, 136, 140,
    149, 180, 181, 183, 230,
    233
free range poultry, 70
frequency modulation, 87
fungi/fungus, 18, 59, 76, 132,
    145, 191, 192, 195
fungicides, 132

G

gait disturbances, 184
galactosamine, 172
gall, 149
gamma
    linolenic, 139
    rays, 65
garlic, 26, 203, 228, 234, 236
gene
    BRCA1 tumor suppressor,
        77
    expression, 64
    p21, 131
    p53 tumor suppressor, 63
genetic
    factors, 38
    instability, 88
    predisposition, 62
    testing, 77
genistein, 96
germ theory, 37
Germanium Sesquioxide, 241
Germany, 146, 157, 165,
    217, 245, 246
Geronimo Rubio, 16, 90
Gerson Therapy, 87, 90, 217,
    218
Gingko Biloba, 236
ginseng, 96, 146, 239
GLA, 222

glioblastoma multiforme, 176
glucuronides, 171
glutamine, 96, 233
glutathione, 108, 126, 127,
    131, 172, 173, 233
    glutathione peroxidase,
        108, 126
glycemic Index, 223
glycolysis, 131
Golden Seal, 146
gonads, 190
gonorrhea, 147
gooseberries, 236
grains, 21, 166, 227, 232
grapefruit, 191, 230
grapes, 109, 130, 132, 228,
    231, 234
Greater Celandine, 165
green
    food, 22, 74, 77, 192, 195,
        196
    leaf juice, 218
    leafy vegetables, 22, 77,
        216, 225, 227, 229
green blue algae, 25, 195
Green Tea, 25, 96, 130, 131,
    183
growth hormone, 36
guar gum, 197, 203, 204

H

H. pylori, 191
Halstead Theory of Cancer,
    81
Harry Hoxsey, 154
Harvard Nurse Study, 70
HDL cholesterol, 13
health indicators, 32
healthcare, 80
heart
    irregular beat, 147
heat-shock proteins, 95
heavy metal, 67, 68, 75, 97,
    100, 117, 189, 196,
    201-203, 210, 214, 215
hemorrhage, 141
hemorrhoids, 147, 180
Hepatitis B, 74, 147
herbal tea, 153, 211, 216
herbicide residues, 65
herpes, 44, 146, 147, 150,
    166
herpes I and II, 147

hair loss, 45
higher-fat, 228
Hiroki Nanba, 159
histamine, 239
histocompatibility complex II, 117
HIV, 147, 166, 191
holistic clinics, 157, 166
holotransferrin, 182
homeopathy, 99, 145
homeostasis, 11, 36, 78, 227
homocysteine, 37
honey, 191
hormone, 19, 23, 70, 77, 82, 87, 190, 201
    balanced profile, 23
    enhancement, 216
    growth, 36
    imbalance, 15, 19, 82, 91
    influences, 38
    metabolism, 64
    pro-aging, 168
    replacement therapy, 69, 70
Hospital Santa Monica, 241
Hoxsey herbs, 154, 155
HRT, 69, 70
human
    fibrosarcoma, 118
    papilloma virus, 74, 191
hyaluronidase, 118
hydrochloric acid, 74
hydrogen peroxide, 21, 107-109, 111, 119, 181, 183, 210, 230, 241
    infusion therapy, 241
    therapy, 21, 181
hydrolysis, 171
hypercalcemia, 175
hyperglycemia, 175
hypertension, 19, 33, 36-38, 160, 161, 175
hyperthermia, 18, 23, 87, 112, 131, 226, 238, 239, 243
hyperthyroidism, 140
hypomagnesaemia, 140
hypothesis, 35, 36, 81, 191
hypothyroidism, 35
Hz, 64

I

IgA, 69, 144
IgD, 144

IgE, 144
IgG, 144
IgM, 144
IL1, 159
immune
    evasion, 88
    stimulator, 177
immune system, 228
immune-compromised, 59
Immunity, 19, 25, 39, 49, 50, 60, 85, 93, 94, 95, 98, 99, 108, 116, 118, 125, 143, 144, 145, 163, 164, 166, 168, 176, 196, 230, 238, 247
immuno-competence, 141
immunoglobulin, 144, 233
Immunoglobulin A, 69
impotence, 163
in vitro, 118, 126, 177, 185
incubation, 70, 182
indictables, 87
industrial
    plants, 226
    toxins, 38, 67
infection, 26, 31, 59, 145, 147, 148, 180, 227, 245
inflammation, 19, 151, 173, 242
inflammatory econsinoids, 156
influenza, 151
Inositol Hexaphosphate, 166
insomnia, 161
insulin, 36, 87, 208, 222, 243
    induced chemotherapy, 87
    potentiation therapy, 243
    resistance, 222
interferon, 163, 194, 196
Interleukin-1 and 2, 161
internal terrain, 12, 15, 18, 38, 39, 49, 76, 77, 82, 187, 193
interstitial
    collagen, 18
intestinal
    flora, 191
    toxicity, 73
    tract, 74, 195
    disorders, 146
intracellular
    makeup, 15
    mutational changes, 107
intravenous, 119, 122, 123, 205, 215, 241

drip, 123
iodine, 155
ion transportation, 140
IP-6, 166, 167
iron
    binding, 233
    modulating protein, 233
    overload, 123
    rich, 181
Iscador, 157
isoprenyl chemical subunits, 136
Israel, 66

J

Jaakkola, 91
jacuzzi, 210
Japan, 32, 121, 228
juice, 23, 208
    celery, 208
Julian Whitaker, 39, 48

K

Karen Lasser, 31
Karl Folkers, 138
kawaratake, 158
Kelley Anti-cancer Therapy, 81
kidney, 18, 47, 71, 118, 123, 149, 154, 155, 167, 172, 200, 203-206, 217, 229, 231
    cleansing, 206
    damage, 45
    stones, 149, 167

L

lactating, 154
lactobacillus acidophilus, 194, 195
lactobacillus bulgaricus, 195
Lactoferrin, 166, 233
Laetrile, 87, 235, 236
LAPd, 128
laxative, 123, 150
LDL-cholesterols, 108
lead, 22, 38, 42, 62, 65, 67, 68, 75, 76, 78, 86, 88, 106-108, 124, 129, 141, 142, 154, 172, 190, 202, 203, 210, 211, 215, 232
leaded gasoline, 202

legumes, 22, 72, 166, 197, 216, 229, 230, 232
lemon juice, 208, 230
lentils, 229, 231
Lentinan, 158
lesions, 228
lethargic, 36
lettuce, 191, 208, 230
leukocytes, 146
lifespan, 13, 91, 221
lifestyle, 11, 38, 62, 75, 80, 87, 102, 104, 168, 216, 246
life-threatening, 41, 48, 92, 98
light beam generator, 242
lima beans, 229, 231
Ling Zhi-8, 161
linseed, 211
Linus Pauling, 84, 117-119, 179, 220
lipase, 193
lipid peroxides, 108
lipoprotein(a), 37
lipoproteins, 107
liquid, 23, 154, 175, 211
    cartilage, 175
    shark cartilage, 175
liver, 9, 18, 23, 46, 74, 75, 94, 117, 132, 151, 157, 159-161, 163, 167, 168, 171-173, 185, 186, 191, 200, 203, 209, 217, 218, 226, 242
    enzymes, 117
    function, 23, 75, 185
    herbs, 217
    toxins, 203
L-lysine, 24, 171, 178
longevity, 23, 133, 144, 162, 163, 246
long-term therapy, 83, 121
Louis Pasteur, 37, 76, 187
low-glycemic
    fruits, 22, 232
    index, 21, 224, 229
L-proline, 24, 171, 178, 179
lumps, 26, 39, 245
lung, 9, 14, 18, 40, 46, 47, 69, 91, 96, 111, 114, 116, 127, 129, 149, 157, 163, 164, 166, 200, 206, 217
    cleansing, 206
    disease, 163, 164
    edema, 127
lupus, 203, 218
lutein, 108

lycopene, 108, 235
lymph
    nodes, 56, 57, 137, 138, 156
    system, 144
lymphatic
    cleansing, 212
    drainage, 212, 243
    drainage machines, 212
    massage, 212
    therapy, 242
lymphoblastic leukemic
    human cell line, 118
lymphocytes, 73, 144, 196
    T4, 146
lymphocytic functions, 140
lymphoid neoplasm, 118
lymphomas, 157, 236

M

macrobiotic diets, 87
macrophages, 108, 137, 145, 156, 215
magnesium, 24, 89, 136, 140, 141, 142, 149, 168, 190, 213, 214, 220
    deficiency, 140, 141
    sulfate, 214
magnetic fields, 241, 242
magnetic resonance imaging, 32
magnetic therapy, 99, 241
maintenance, 206, 216
maitake, 25, 131, 158, 159, 160, 161, 164, 176
Maitake Pro-D, 160
mal-absorption syndrome, 74
malaria, 147, 180, 181, 183
male leukemia, 46
malignant tumors, 42, 56
malnutrition, 22, 50, 59, 60, 136, 220, 221
mammary glands, 132
mammogram, 65
mammography, 46, 59, 138, 139
manganese, 107, 109
margarine, 229
matrix, 18, 24, 175, 177-179
Max Gerson, 217
Mayo Clinic, 120
mechanism
    compensatory, 36
    regulatory, 61

medical
    diagnosis, 20, 103
    mushroom, 25, 164
    science, 14, 37, 40
Medical College of Wisconsin, 68
medicinal mushroom, 74, 87, 152, 158, 164
meditation, 73, 87
mega-dose, 91
megavitamin, 179
mega-vitamin, 91
melanoma, 46, 47, 60, 63, 90, 112, 116, 118, 126, 166, 182, 218, 226
    cell growth, 112, 226
melatonin, 64, 89, 95, 96
membrane, 107, 126, 128, 149, 184, 222, 238
    chorioallantoic, 177
meningitis, 147
menopause, 36, 69
    anxiety, 161
menstruating, 69
    irregularities, 146
mental condition, 243
mercury, 22, 67, 129, 202, 215
    fillings, 67
meridians, 99
metabolic
    dysfunction, 15, 82
    hyperthermia, 18
metabolism
    high, 86
metalo-vitamin, 183
metals, 23, 201, 202, 214, 215
metamucil, 211
metastases, 57, 82
metastasis, 15, 88, 93, 94, 123, 166
metastatic growth, 15, 81
methionine, 203
Mexico, 12, 16, 90, 166, 238, 244, 246
MHC II, 117
microbes, 59, 76, 107, 203
microbial toxins, 203
micronutrient, 110-114
microwave ovens, 63, 64
migraine, 217
milk thistle, 23, 75, 171, 172, 203
millet, 191, 223, 227, 229
mineral ascorbates, 178

minerals, 23, 27, 87, 96, 109, 128, 139, 150, 189, 190, 193, 195, 206, 213, 218, 220, 247
Mistletoe, 87
mitomycin, 156, 159
mitotic cell cycle, 131
modalities, 10, 34, 41, 46, 49, 52, 92, 97, 99, 122, 238, 246
Monomorphism Theory, 76
mouse
  ascites tumor cells, 118
  lymphocytic leukemia cells, 118
  sarcoma cells, 118
mucous, 150
  producing foods, 74
mulberries, 132
multi-drug resistance, 95
muscle strength, 22, 129
mushroom polysaccharides, 95
mustard gas, 41
mutagenic properties, 42
mutational
  changes, 19, 38, 50, 86, 106, 136
  damage, 24, 63, 84
myasthenia gravis, 204
myeloma, 30

N

NAC, 115
N-acetylcysteine, 115
National Academy of Science, 67
National Cancer Institute, 34, 41, 68, 149, 150, 220
natural compounds, 10, 11, 17, 27, 48, 49, 86, 88, 89, 94, 95, 106, 136, 170, 171, 173, 238, 247
natural medicine, 10-13, 15, 19, 21, 22, 29, 48, 49, 51, 54, 78-82, 85-87, 92, 100, 101, 104, 154, 169, 246
  vs. conventional medicine, 48
  arsenal, 87
natural resonant frequencies, 64

natural therapy, 11, 53, 54, 86, 92, 93, 94, 237
natural-oriented, 10, 26, 80-82, 93, 106, 112, 122, 245
necrosis, 123, 193
nectarines, 229, 231
negative polarity, 242
negative side effects, 17, 94, 95, 155
nervousness, 211
Netherlands, 223, 245, 246
neurotoxic symptoms, 181
neurotransmitters, 74
niacin, 192
niacinamide, 25, 142
nickel, 67, 202
nicotine, 205
nitrogen, 22, 183, 233
nitrogenous waste, 71
nitrosamines, 71, 117
NK, 69
Nobel laureate, 84, 117, 179
nodes, 57
nodular masses, 151
non-localized breast cancer, 14, 40
non-sedating, 31
non-toxic, 9-12, 16, 18, 24, 41, 45, 48, 49, 54, 80, 87-89, 94, 97, 104, 106, 116, 128, 133, 165, 171, 176, 221, 238, 241, 246
  polynucleotide reductase, 128
Nordic-Germanic ancestry, 232
nucleic magnesium depletion, 141
nucleus, 88, 106, 136, 177, 196
nutrition, 15, 18, 22, 23, 25, 38, 48-52, 58, 71, 81, 87, 91, 107, 112-116, 128, 136, 138, 155, 168, 178, 189, 192, 206-208, 211, 218-221, 225, 228, 232
  absorption, 22, 197
  medicine, 49
  supplements, 39, 72, 87, 92, 183

O

Oasis Hospital, 12, 16, 90
oat bran, 197, 203, 204
oats, 223, 229
obesity, 39, 210
OH groups, 178
OH-ions, 188
Ojibwa native tribe, 148
old-age diseases, 151, 218
Oleuropein, 147
oligoglucan, 161
olive leaf, 147, 148
oncogenes, 77
  activation, 64
oncogenic viruses, 118
oncology, 12, 13, 27, 50, 81, 91, 247
  oncologists, 30, 91, 200
onions, 109, 130, 131, 228, 234
organic
  buttermilk, 231
  depression, 146
  low-fat cottage cheese, 231
  whole foods, 22
  yogurt, 231
organism, 61, 77, 78, 81, 181
organochlorine pesticides, 117
organs, 56, 63, 66, 86, 99, 144, 149, 150, 177, 200, 205, 208
orthomolecular, 12, 27, 50, 247
osteoporosis, 71
Otto Warburg, 75
ovary, 23, 91
overhead lights, 63
over-the-counter douches, 67
oxygen, 15, 17, 21, 58, 60, 69, 75, 76, 81, 83, 86, 107, 108, 126, 128, 136, 137, 181, 188-190, 208, 212, 222, 233, 235, 240, 241
  atoms, 240
  hyperbaric, 87, 240
  intermediates, 233
  singlet, 108, 235
oxygenate, 21

oxygen-generating modalities, 21
ozonated water bath, 230
ozone, 21, 63, 87, 210, 241
  insuflation, 240

P

p53, 63, 69, 131, 167
palladium, 128
  complex, 128
palliative treatment, 44
pancreas, 9, 46, 175
pantethine mixed, 25
parasites, 18, 58, 61, 74, 192, 213
parsley, 109, 130, 191, 208, 230
parsnip, 231
pastas, 222
pasteurized, 37
pathogenic, 76
Patrick Quillin, 219, 220
Paul Allen, 31
peaches, 191, 229, 231
peanuts, 77, 132, 191, 233
penicillin, 180
Penn State University, 162
peppermint leaf, 216
pepsin, 74
peptic ulcer
  asymptomatic, 123
peripheral nerve injury, 45
peritoneal macrophages, 163
pesticide, 65, 66, 202
PET scans, 97
pH, 22, 188-191, 213, 214
phagocytic activities, 118
phagocytosis, 163, 242
pharmaceutical industry, 43
photoluminotescence, 240
physical activity, 22
phytoalexins, 173
phytoestrogen, 235
pineapple, 191, 229
placebo, 120, 122, 125
plant oils, 71
plasma ascorbate levels, 119
plastics, 70
platelet aggregation, 172, 240
plums, 229
pneumonia, 48, 147
poison, 9, 14, 41, 53, 177, 218, 245

pollution, 17, 38, 106, 107, 220
polycyclic hydrocarbons, 117
Polydox, 128
Polymorphism Theory, 76
Poly-MVA, 128-130, 183
polysaccharide, 150, 158, 162-164, 176
poor dietary habit, 19
pork, 154
positive polarity, 242
post-menopausal, 140
potassium, 154, 155, 213, 218, 230
potassium iodide, 154, 155
potato, 21, 72, 73, 222, 225, 231
powdered lignite, 214
powdered shark cartilage, 89, 174
powered supplementation, 25
praseodymium nitrate, 172
pregnant, 42, 147, 154, 175
premenopausal, 228
preneoplastic lesions, 132
preservatives, 66, 226
prevention, 37, 80, 85, 86, 113, 117, 122, 129, 132, 133, 167
prickly ash bark, 154
prions, 18
proanthocyanidins, 109, 130
probiotics, 22, 74, 77, 97, 191, 192, 194, 195, 211
pro-carcinogens, 234
processed food, 17, 71
progesterone, 13, 69, 70, 125
  deficiency, 69
prognosis, 20, 58, 103
prognostic Factors, 57
programmed cell death, 172
proline, 178
pro-oxidant, 111
prophylactic, 77, 86, 141
  mastectomy, 77
Propulsid, 32
prostaglandin, 173
prostaglandin E2, 156
prostate marker, 160
protein, 18, 87, 88, 108, 128, 140, 192, 195, 196, 204, 229-233, 239, 240
  by-product toxins, 201
  C reactive, 185

calorie malnutrition, 220
cell-wall deficient, 76
plant, 229
plant-based, 22, 72
proteoglycan, 177
protocol, 10, 24, 52, 94, 124
protozoans, 147
PSA, 160, 233
PSK, 95, 158
psoriasis, 147, 203
PSP, 95
psychiatrist, 99
psychotherapy, 98
psyllium, 197, 203, 217
  husk powder, 217
  seeds, 203
pulse, 191, 243
pumpkin, 231
pureed carrots, 229

Q

qigong, 87, 99
qinghaosu, 180
quercetin, 25, 96, 131, 239
quinone chemical group, 136

R

radiation
  exposure, 44
radiation therapy, 9, 14, 34, 41, 44, 45, 85, 114, 120, 140, 185, 236, 241
radio waves, 239
radioactive particles, 68
radionuclides, 68
radon, 69
raisin, 191, 231
Ralph Moss, 43, 237
raspberries, 236
raw materials, 216
RDA, 24, 91, 113, 140, 141, 220
reactive chemical particles, 17
recrudescent rate, 181
rectal, 60, 68
rectum, 46, 71, 240
red
  clover, 152, 154
  meat, 71, 77, 190, 227
  peel, 216
redundancy, 89

Reishi Mushroom, 131, 160, 161, 164
relapse, 176
religion, 99
remission, 9, 11, 13, 30, 85, 113, 147, 176, 183, 185, 206, 219, 235
renal functions, 163
Rene Caisse, 148, 149
resonance, 99, 182
respiratory tract, 164
response rate, 43, 180, 239, 247
resveratrol, 132, 168, 171, 173
reticulocyte count, 184, 185
reticuloendothelial system, 163
retroviruses, 147
reversal rate, 16, 90
reverse osmosis, 213
rhamnogalacturonan, 198
rhein, 150
rhinitis, 127
riboflavin, 192
Rife Technology, 23, 239
risk
    factors, 38, 56, 62, 69, 77, 78
    reduction, 63-65, 67-70, 72-77
Rudy Falk, 129
rye, 229

S

saliva, 190
salmonella, 192
Samuel Epstein, 52
sarcoma, 141, 157, 236
sarcoma-37 systems, 150
sauna bath, 209
saw palmetto, 180
Schizophyllan, 158
screening tool, 37, 47
scurvy, 113, 124
sea salt, 210, 227
secondary cigarette smoke, 201
sedentary, 38, 62
seeds, 216, 227, 229, 235
Seldane, 31
selenium, 24, 95, 109, 114, 126, 127, 139, 149, 168
self-administer, 89

self-cleansing, 205
self-healing, 205
senna leaf, 216
serum
    albumin, 220
    ascorbate, 122
sesame, 231
severely depressed, 50
sexual organs, 66
shallow breathing, 76
shark cartilage, 171, 174-177
Sheep Sorrel, 150, 152
shingles, 147
shitake, 25, 158, 162, 164
Siberian Ginseng, 146
sickness, 35, 76
side effects, 31, 42, 44, 82, 85, 88, 96, 115, 123, 126, 129, 132, 157, 160, 165, 175, 176, 184, 242, 243, 246
sigmoid colonic cancer, 163
Signs of Cancer, 60
silent killer, 37, 222
silymarin, 97, 172, 173
skin, 18, 42, 56, 60, 63, 118, 127, 132, 150, 151, 154, 155, 172, 175, 194, 200, 203, 206, 208-211, 217
    brushing, 209
    cleansing, 206, 208, 209
    irritations, 42
Slippery Elm, 149, 152
small intestine damage, 156
smoking, 38, 69
smoking-related, 69
SOD, 115
sodium ascorbate, 119, 123
sodium silicate, 214
solar radiation, 63
soluble fiber, 204
solvents, 203
sorrel, 149, 150
soy, 109, 191, 227, 232-234
    products, 191, 234
spinach, 208, 225, 227, 229, 230
spirulina, 25, 195, 196
spleen, 194
spontaneous
    regression, 92
    remission, 221
sprays, 202, 226
sprouted
    seeds, 191

squash, 227, 231
stage, 16, 20, 36, 56, 57, 85, 90, 99, 103, 123, 138, 170, 171, 210, 211, 239, 247
stage III, 16, 90, 171
staphylococcus, 192
starving cancer cell, 21
Stephen Sinatra, 105
steria leaf, 216
stillingia root, 154
stimulant, 130
stomach, 56, 60, 71, 122, 151, 153, 157, 160, 191, 194, 236
    disorders, 146
    ulcers, 151
stone fruits, 235
streptococci, 166
streptococcus faecium, 195
stress, 17, 38, 61, 73, 87, 95, 99, 168, 216, 223, 230, 232
    oxidative, 49, 108, 233
    reduction, 87, 99, 216
stroke, 19, 35, 141, 167, 172
structural functionality, 38
sub-clinically malnourished, 220
sublingual, 142
submicroscopic dysfunctional causes, 15
suehirotake, 158
sugar, 17, 21, 36, 58, 71, 77, 83, 128, 136, 137, 149, 161, 196, 205, 207, 208, 221-223, 225-227, 230, 243
    feeder, 21
    high, 19, 207, 223, 228
    imbalance, 36
    intake, 21, 223
    low, 21, 86, 223
    refined, 21, 72, 222
sulfated castor oil, 214
sulfur, 154
sunflower, 231
sunscreens, 63
Super Oxide Dismutase, 107
support group, 23, 73, 102
suppositories, 88
surgery, 9, 14, 26, 31, 34, 41, 44, 45, 59, 80, 82, 83, 93, 98, 139, 151, 175, 245
surgical excision, 41

sweating, 144, 209
sweet potato, 231
Switzerland, 157, 245, 246
symptom
    allergy, 157
    alleviation, 33
    localized, 15, 81
    outward, 36, 37
    relief, 37
synergistic cytotoxic effect,
    17, 95
synthetic DNA reductase, 128
systemic
    disease, 15, 33, 34, 81
    poisoning, 61
    weakening, 59

T

tablets, 25, 88, 125, 164, 194
talc, 154
Tamoxifen, 70, 126
tangeretin, 115, 131, 132
tap water, 68, 210, 213, 226
tastes, 48, 208
T-cell proliferation, 156
T-cells, 117, 158, 161, 193
tea, 77, 109, 130, 148, 149,
    151-154, 211, 216, 227
technology, 14, 32, 39, 40,
    49, 246
temperature
    body, 18, 155, 157, 238
    high, 18, 58, 86
    sensitive, 18
terfenadine, 31
terminal cancer, 16, 90, 121,
    123, 189
tertiary amine, 183
testicles, 60
The Cancer Industry, 43, 237
T-helper cells, 145
therapeutic tool, 50
therapy, 10-13, 16, 17, 23,
    26, 30, 34, 39, 41, 45-49,
    51, 52, 54, 60, 80, 82-85,
    87, 89-91, 93, 94, 97, 98,
    100, 106, 111, 122, 133,
    200, 221, 238, 241,
    245-247
    combination, 16, 92
    oxygenating, 87, 240
    ozone, 87, 241
thiamin, 192

Thiotepa, 165
thyme, 109, 130
thymus, 73, 157, 168, 194
    gland, 73, 157
thyroid
    disorders, 151
    gland, 155
    hormone levels, 36
TIBC, 185
tissue
    connective, 170, 236
    epithelial, 170
    non-cancerous, 66
    extracts, 87
T-lymphocytes, 145, 162, 198
tobacco, 62, 68, 69, 75, 76,
    227
tocopherol radicals, 127
tomatoes, 154, 228, 231, 235
tonic, 154, 161-164
toxic,
    buildup, 52, 86
    chemicals, 22, 66, 67,
        172, 201, 204, 233
    metal cleansing, 206, 214
    metals, 202
    necrosis, 127
    overload, 45
toxicity, 42, 48, 83, 95, 116,
    129, 137, 165, 181, 183,
    185, 200, 202, 230
toxin, 18, 22, 191, 200, 201,
    202, 207, 216
    amanita, 172
    clearance mechanism, 18
    secretion, 191
trace minerals, 138, 213
trans-fat, 19, 71, 72
Transition Phase of aging, 35
transplant rejections, 161
tremors, 202
triglyceride, 13, 223
T-suppressor cells, 145
tuberculosis, 147, 217
Tulane University, 92
tumeric, 25
tumor, 11, 15, 37, 42, 43,
    49, 57-61, 66, 68, 69,
    73, 77, 81, 82, 90, 91,
    93, 118-120, 123, 126,
    129-133, 139, 141, 145,
    149-151, 156, 157, 159,
    161, 162, 170, 171, 173,
    185, 189, 193, 208, 228,
    239, 240, 241, 247

benign, 18, 59
    hemorrhage, 123
    hormone-sensitive, 152
    malignant, 42, 56
    mammary, 118, 222
    markers, 37, 185
    multiplicity, 171
    regression, 130, 139
Turkey Rhubarb Root, 150,
    152
turnip tops, 191

U

Ukrain, 87, 165, 166
ulceration, 97
ulcerative colitis, 203
ultraviolet,
    blood irradiation, 240
    B and C radiation, 63
umbilical endothelial cells,
    174
under-active thyroids, 155
University of California, 65, 79
University of Maryland, 167
University of Texas, 138
unsaturated oils, 229
unsulfured dried fruits, 236
upper pharynx, 74
urinary
    bleeding, 60
    pH Test, 190
urine pH, 191
uterine, 47, 60, 125, 235
uterus, 23, 71, 91
uva ursi leaf, 216

V

vaginal discharge, 60
variance, 20, 103
vascular endothelial growth
    factor, 174
vegetable, 23, 196, 206-208,
    222, 225, 229-231
    cruciferous, 235
    fresh juices, 23
    hydrogenated oil, 71
    juice, 206, 208
    juicing, 206
    raw, 229
    vegetarian, 92, 216, 232
    vegetarianism, 87
vibrational energy, 99
vibratory frequencies, 239

Victor A Marcial-Vega, 143
Vincent Speckhart, 33
vincristine, 156
vinegar, 154, 227
visualization, 87
vitamin
    A, 24, 91, 96, 114, 116,
       149, 220, 235
    B, 24, 91, 128, 136, 142,
       220, 235
    B6, 192
    B12, 24, 142, 220
    B17, 235
    B9, 24
    C, 24, 30, 53, 69, 84,
       91, 95, 96, 108, 109,
       111-114, 117-125,
       127, 130, 131, 138,
       151, 154, 160, 161,
       169, 171, 172, 178,
       179, 183, 220, 221,
       225, 241
    C deficiency, 221
    E, 24, 25, 91, 95-97, 108,
       109, 112, 125-127,
       138-140, 185, 226
    E succinate, 112, 126,
       226
    supplement, 91
Vitamin C and Cancer, 53,
    91, 151

W

W.S. Halstead, 81
wakame miso soup, 191
warfarin, 147
Wassyl J. Nowicky, 165
water, 24, 38, 66-68, 71, 72,
    108, 124, 127, 128, 130,
    152, 153, 182, 184,
    195-198, 200, 202, 204,
    208, 210-214, 216, 217,
    226, 227, 229, 230, 241
    bottled, 213
    distilled, 152, 213
    mineral, 190, 191, 214
    pollutants, 226
    pure filtered, 23, 68, 77,
       213
waxes, 226
weakness, 44, 60, 182
well-being, 23, 52, 80, 102,
    113, 119, 140, 195, 235
wheat grass, 25, 195

whey protein, 233
white blood cells, 56, 107,
    117, 144, 145, 146, 148,
    215
white bread, 222, 224
whole grain
    bread, 197, 229
    tortilla, 229
whole wheat, 190
whole-body, 239
    phenomenon, 15, 81
withdrawals, 31
World Health Organization,
    32, 35, 72, 201
wrinkles, 35

X

xenoestrogens, 67
X-ray, 65, 77

Y

yam, 231
yeast tablets, 154
yellow powder, 154

Z

zeaxanthin, 108, 235
zinc, 13, 24, 91, 107, 109,
    127, 154, 168
zinc chloride, 154
zoetron Therapy, 243